EVALUATION OF LIVER FUNCTION

in Clinical Practice

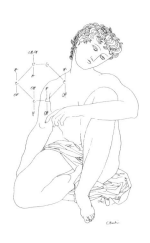

Published by THE LILLY RESEARCH LABORATORIES

Indianapolis, Indiana

PREPARED BY

Carroll M. Leevy, M.D., F.A.C.P.
Professor of Medicine
Seton Hall College of Medicine
Jersey City, New Jersey

EDITORIAL CONSULTANTS

Hans Popper, M.D., F.A.C.P.
Director of Pathology
Mount Sinai Hospital
New York, New York

Charles S. Davidson, M.D., F.A.C.P.
Associate Professor of Medicine
Harvard Medical School
Boston, Massachusetts

PUBLISHED BY

The Lilly Research Laboratories
Indianapolis, Indiana

S. O. Waife, M.D., F.A.C.P.
Assistant Director
Medical Research Division

C. E. Hammond
Senior Art Director

EVALUATION OF LIVER FUNCTION

in Clinical Practice

Contents

Evaluation of Liver Function in Clinical Practice

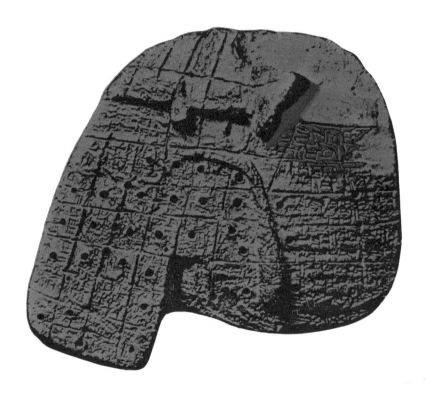

Figure 1. Clay model of a sheep's liver, used in Babylonia about 2000 B.C. (British Museum).

1

Introduction

"For the king of Babylon stood at the parting of the way,
at the head of the two ways, to use divination:
he made his arrows bright, he consulted with images,
<u>*he looked in the liver.*"</u>

—*Ezekiel 21:21*

In the days of Babylonia, the priest-physician would examine minutely the liver of sacrificial animals for signs of import from the gods (divination). In fact, the earliest known anatomic sculpture is a clay model of a sheep's liver with a divinatory text dating from about 2000 B.C. (Figure 1). The liver was chosen because it contains the most blood; since life and blood are synonymous, the liver was considered the seat of the soul.

Throughout much of recorded history there was a belief that the liver was in the center of things, which, in truth, it is. Consider the theory of the four humors—buried in the teachings of Hippocrates, Empedocles, and Aristotle. ". . . blood is hot and moist like air, phlegm is cold and moist like water, yel-low bile is hot and dry like fire, and black bile is cold and dry like earth. As one or other of these humors predominated in an individual, he was supposed to be of a sanguine, phlegmatic, choleric, or melancholy temperament."[1] Note that Shakespeare followed this concept in *Julius Caesar*, in which Mark Antony is sanguine, Octavius phlegmatic, Cassius choleric, and Brutus melancholic.

This idea did not die with the advent of modern science. Indeed, a mere century ago, in the writings of one of the great founders of modern pathology, Karl von Rokitansky (1804-1878), there is a strong espousal of the humoral concept.[2] (It was Rudolf Virchow who administered the *coup de grâce*.)

Although these misconceptions were partly

dispelled with the inauguration of the age of experimental medicine, the liver has many mysteries and unexplored aspects which continue to intrigue man.

The practicing physician still faces as major clinical problems the recognition of hepatic disease, assessment of its etiology, severity, and activity, and evaluation of hepatic regenerative capacity. The clinician's work has been facilitated by the development of numerous clinical and laboratory methods which permit a study of its morphologic, biochemical, and physiologic status.

The value of various laboratory procedures in the diagnosis and treatment of liver disease has often been emphasized. However, no single test provides an over-all picture of the functional state of the liver. This is understandable, for in one sense the liver is several organs in one. It consists of a complex circu-

latory system, biliary passages, a collection of reticuloendothelial cells of various types, and the "liver cells," or polygonal parenchymal cells themselves (Figure 2a).

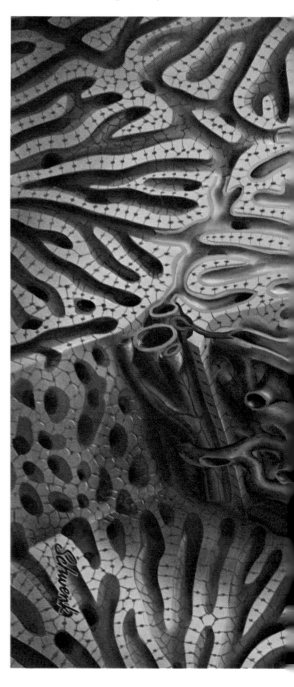

Central vein

Hepatic cells

Biliary canaliculi

Sinusoids

Branch of hepatic artery

Portal area

Branch of portal vein

Bile ducts

Figure 2a. The liver lobule. Artist's rendition of the structure of the liver showing the vascular, biliary, and parenchymal structures.

Interference with the functions of one or more of these physiologic–anatomic components is responsible for the clinical and laboratory abnormalities found in liver disease. Moreover, an evaluation of the functional reserve of the individual systems provides an insight into the extent and nature of the pathologic process.

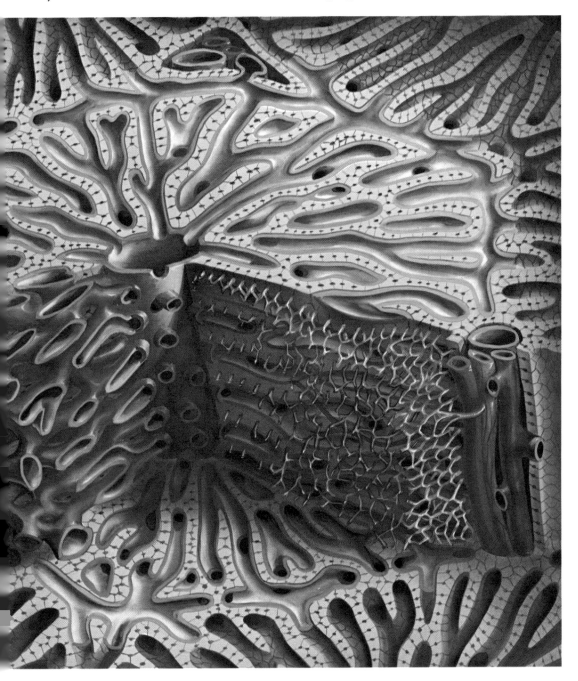

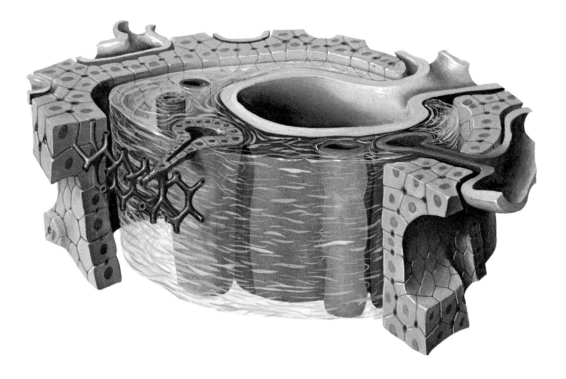

PHYSIOLOGIC-ANATOMIC UNITS OF THE LIVER

The liver consists of four discrete but interrelated structures which are physiologic-anatomic units. Considered in this light, they will aid considerably in the practical application of our knowledge of the liver.

Circulatory System—The liver is unique in that it has a dual blood supply consisting of the hepatic artery and portal vein, both of which participate in the transport of oxygen and foodstuffs to this organ for assimilation. Sinusoids surrounding the liver cells merge to form central veins which empty into sublobular veins, large collecting veins, then into the hepatic veins, and finally into the inferior vena cava. The blood vessels are accompanied by lymphatics and nerve fibers. Lymph channels carry liver lymph with its high protein

Figure 2b. Detail of a portal area.

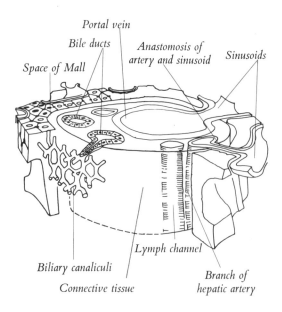

content from the liver into the general circulation and aid in the transport of material from the splanchnic bed to the systemic circulation (Figure 2b). Nerve fibers transmit sensory impulses and help regulate intrasinusoidal vascular pressure and blood flow.

Biliary Passages — The biliary passages consist of a series of thin-walled tubes into which conjugated bilirubin, cholesterol, certain drugs, and other substances are secreted by the liver cells. Within the liver cell, the system originates with the Golgi apparatus, which consists of lamellae and vesicles adjacent to microvilli of the bile canaliculi lying between liver cells. Bile canaliculi represent the biliary cell wall or plasma membrane of the liver cells. They empty into bile ductules which, in turn, lead to interlobular bile ducts (small), septal bile ducts (medium), large intrahepatic bile ducts, and, finally, main branches of the common bile duct.

Reticuloendothelial Cells — The reticuloendothelial system is widely distributed; however, 60 percent of its elements are found in the liver, 5 percent consist of reticular cells in the spleen, and the remaining 35 percent are present in the lymph nodes and other tissues. Reticuloendothelial, or "sinusoidal," cells in the liver are of three varieties: 25 percent protrude as stellate phagocytic (Kupffer) cells (Figure 2c), 50 percent are flat phagocytic cells, and 25 percent are endothelial cells.

Parenchymal Cells — Parenchymal cells are the liver cells which take a polyhedral form after fixation and are contiguous to sinusoids on one side; the other surface area is enmeshed by bile capillaries. These cells vary in diameter between 18 and 30 microns and contain a nucleus and a cytoplasm which is rich in such structures as mitochondria, endoplasmic

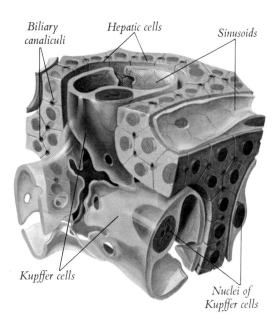

Figure 2c. Kupffer cells lining the hepatic sinusoid.

reticula, lysosomes, and inclusions (described later, see page 43, Figure 15). Liver cells maintain a constant interchange with the vascular and biliary systems. Those situated around the terminal afferent vascular branches receive more oxygen and nutrients than those peripheral to this area. It was originally thought that afferent vessels terminated around the portal area; however, studies by Rappaport[3] suggest that they end in an area called the "acinus," which is located between the central vein and the portal area. At any rate, the traditional view of the liver lobule as a hexagonal unit is being changed as research continues. "Thus, to speak of hexagonally shaped units in the liver is equivalent to the assumption that there is a regular geometrical pattern in the branched crown of a tree. It may perhaps be closer to reality to consider the liver a biliovascular tree in which the interspaces between the branches are filled with parenchyma."[3]

2

Clinical Recognition of Liver Disease

Liver disease should be suspected in a patient when there is a history of previous jaundice, dietary imbalance, chronic alcoholism, or exposure to known hepatotoxins or when diseases commonly accompanied by liver injury are present. For example, virus hepatitis is suggested by the occurrence of malaise and jaundice six to eight weeks after receipt of a whole-blood transfusion; cirrhosis is probably present in most alcoholics with poor dietary intake who develop jaundice, ascites, and hematemesis; liver abscess is the most probable cause in a patient with fever and pain in the scapula and liver area as a complication of amebic dysentery.

A careful physical examination remains the single most important method for detecting liver disease and following its course. Frequently, there are gross alterations in the structure of the organ, such as enlargement or atrophy of the liver as a whole or of one of its lobes; or there may be changes in its tex-

ture, such as an increase in its softness, hardness, or nodularity. In addition, there may be tenderness or spontaneous pain. Liver injury itself may lead to secondary disturbances elsewhere, which may be manifested by jaundice, spider angiomas, splenomegaly, bleeding esophageal varices, peripheral edema, ascites, fetor, or mental disturbances.

Changes in the position and size of the liver usually are readily recognizable on physical examination. This is best achieved by measurement of the anterior linear projection of the organ *from the upper border of relative dullness* to its palpable edge in the midclavicular and midsternal line. Normal values depend upon body habitus; for example, in a hyposthenic individual, the right midclavicular linear projection has a tendency to be longer than that found in a mesomorph or hypersthenic individual (Figure 3). Measurements reveal that the average male has an over-all anterior linear projection in the midclavicular line of 15 ± 2 cm. and in the midsternal line of 4 ± 1 cm.[4] Such measurements provide an excellent correlation with liver size as determined by photoscans and postmortem studies (Figure 4).

It should be noted that measurement of the degree that the liver extends below the costal margin shows *no* correlation with actual size (Figure 5), for emphysema or other chest diseases may cause its downward displacement,

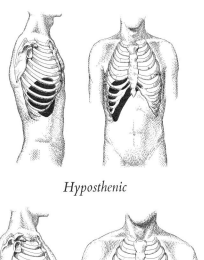

Hyposthenic

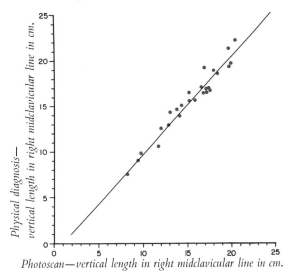

Figure 4. Correlation of linear surface projection as determined by means of physical examination and photoscans. (Reproduced by permission[4])

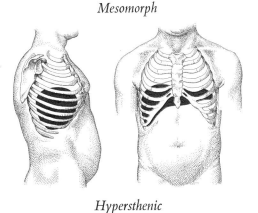

Mesomorph

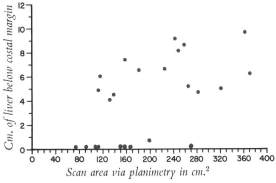

Figure 5. Lack of correlation of liver projection below thoracic cage as determined by physical examination and anterior surface projection established by photoscans. (Reproduced by permission[4])

Hypersthenic

Figure 3. Body habitus and the liver. Anterior and lateral views of the position of the liver in persons with different body configurations.

and selective upward enlargement may not be reflected in subcostal changes. Therefore, the expression "the liver edge is palpable two fingerbreadths below the costal margin" has little meaning. *Photoscans* provide a readily available method for confirming this physical finding (Box 1).

Palpation yields information on the texture

BOX 1
PHOTOSCANS OF THE LIVER

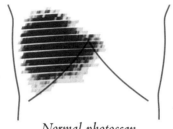

Normal photoscan

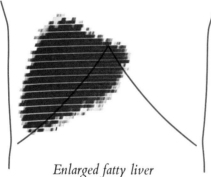

Enlarged fatty liver

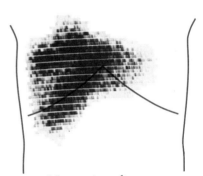

Metastatic malignancy

Photoscans of the liver provide valuable data supplementary to physical examination. They may be employed to give graphic information on posterior and lateral as well as anterior aspects of this organ. Photoscans facilitate the recognition of metastatic malignancy in the liver, aid in the diagnosis and localization of hepatic abscess and parasitic and other cysts, and permit delineation of the size and position of the liver in ascites and other conditions which interfere with physical examination. The procedure is based on the fact that gamma-emitting radioisotopes, such as I^{131} albumin, I^{131} rose bengal, Mo^{99}, and colloidal gold^{198}, are selectively taken up by the liver and concentrate in the parenchymal and reticuloendothelial cells. Of these isotopes, I^{131} rose bengal and Au^{198} are the ones most commonly used; unlike that of I^{131} albumin and Mo^{99}, their hepatic localization allows immediate scanning. I^{131} rose bengal is largely concentrated in the parenchymal hepatic cells, whereas Au^{198} is taken up by the Kupffer cells.

of the liver and on the presence or absence of tenderness. The normal liver has a soft but firm consistency. It initially becomes softer and less consistent with congestion or acute inflammation and becomes more consistent and may progress to rocklike hardness with cirrhosis and neoplastic infiltration. The degree of tenderness depends upon the nature of the hepatic lesion and the amount of pressure exerted by the examiner. A useful point to remember is that a light touch may elicit a painful response in acute congestion (which may be caused by heart failure), liver abscess, metastatic malignancy, or acute hepatitis.

Of course, the most striking aberration which focuses attention on the liver is jaundice. It becomes apparent when the skin and mucous membranes are stained by bile pigments and is usually detectable when the concentration of serum bilirubin reaches about 2 mg. per 100 ml. Artificial light may make recognition of jaundice more difficult; the discoloration must be differentiated from that due to carotenemia (and administration of quinacrine and related drugs). Jaundice, which is often preceded by dark urine or light stools, is most evident in the ocular conjunctivas. It is often accompanied by pruritus and may be associated with xanthoma when it is due to prolonged biliary obstruction.

Bean's classic studies on cutaneous spider angiomas,[5] which are often seen in liver disease, have focused attention on their frequency. These lesions are not specific for liver disease and are often seen in normal pregnancy and other conditions. Nevertheless, they are of considerable diagnostic value when hepatic disease is suspected. These vascular spider angiomas represent minute arteriovenous anastomoses and appear principally on the head, neck, upper thorax, and arms—in the drainage area of the superior vena cava (Figure 6). These structures may be differentiated

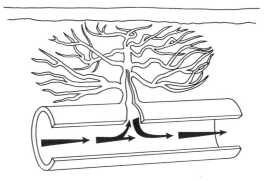

Figure 6. Schematic view of spider angioma showing close connection with cutaneous collecting veins and direction of blood flow.

from other cutaneous lesions by the application and release of pressure with a glass slide.

Splenomegaly, esophageal varices, and ascites are frequently prominent signs of portal hypertension accompanying liver disease. These findings, however, may also be seen in patients with liver disease in the absence of an elevated portal pressure; they are usually directly related to alterations in the intrahepatic circulation.

The reported incidence of clinical enlargement of the spleen in liver disease varies considerably, partly because of difficulty in palpating this retroperitoneal organ. *In-situ* examination is facilitated by placing the patient's left fist under the lower left thorax to bring the spleen forward. One should remember, however, that palpability does not necessarily denote splenic enlargement, for a palpable spleen may not be enlarged, and an enlarged spleen may not be palpable.

Gastro-intestinal bleeding constitutes the most important and devastating complication of liver disease accompanied by portal hypertension. It is due in the majority of instances to rupture of esophageal varices, but it may also occur from a bleeding peptic ulcer or other lesions. The site of hemorrhage can usually be pinpointed by use of a modified "string" test,[6] barium studies of the gastro-intestinal tract, or endoscopy (Box 2).

Ascites, usually associated with muscle wasting, accounts for the typical spiderlike configuration exhibited by many patients with chronic advanced liver disease. It results from a disparity between entry and outflow of fluid from the peritoneal cavity due to a combination of hepatic venous blockade, lym-

---

BOX 2

BLEEDING ESOPHAGEAL VARICES

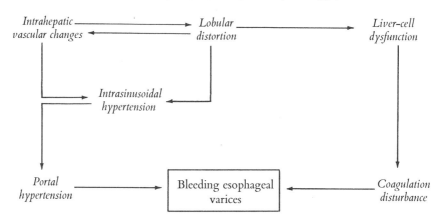

Pathogenesis of bleeding esophageal varices

Esophageal and gastric varices are usually a manifestation of collateral circulation incident to portal hypertension. An elevated portal pressure results when there is interference with the blood's leaving or entering the liver. In chronic liver disease, this most often is caused by distortion of the hepatic lobule or by transmission of hepatic arterial pressure to the portal venous system through intrahepatic arterio-venous shunts. Varices may occur in the lower third of the esophagus in the absence of liver disease or portal hypertension. Rupture of varices may result from a sudden increase in portal pressure or from ulceration of the mucous membrane. Clotting abnormalities help perpetuate bleeding. The fluorescein string test (see page 70) is of great value in determining whether gastro-intestinal hemorrhage is due to a ruptured esophageal varix. In the absence of hemorrhage, esophageal varices (which should be suspected in all patients with chronic liver disease) may be demonstrated by esophagoscopy, splenoportography, and barium studies of the esophagus. Esophagoscopy by an experienced endoscopist offers the most direct and reliable procedure for identifying varices; splenoportography is the next best method in the absence of hemorrhagic tendencies. Barium studies of the esophagus are frequently diagnostic, but the incidence of positive results is related and proportional to the care and technic used. Proper spot filming (performed with the patient in the right anterior oblique position after a thick barium cream was swallowed during the Valsalva maneuver) increases the number of positive esophagrams.

BOX 3

ASCITES

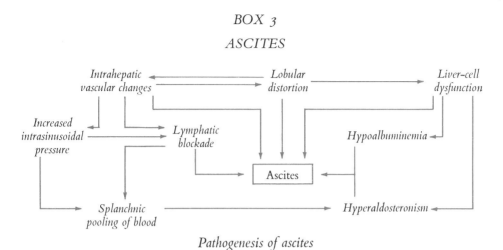

Pathogenesis of ascites

Ascites is one of the major diagnostic and therapeutic problems confronting the physician who cares for patients with chronic liver disease. The first important task is to decide whether the liver disease is responsible; it is usually possible to do so by clinical and laboratory examination. If ascites is due to hepatic disease, identification of the major pathophysiologic alterations responsible for its accumulation is important in deciding treatment and prognosis. The mechanism of ascites is usually complex and includes (1) obstruction to hepatic venous outflow, lymphatic blockage, and portal hypertension; (2) hypoalbuminemia with decreased collateral osmotic pressure; and (3) secondary hyperaldosteronism and increased antidiuretic activity. It would appear that the mechanical factors listed under (1) constitute the most important of these.

CAUSE	PROMINENT CLINICAL FEATURES	PROTEIN CONTENT OF FLUID	SEDIMENT	PORTAL PRESSURE
Cirrhosis	Evidence of liver failure	Transudate	Macrophages	Increased
Metastatic malignancy	Weight loss, evidence of malignancy	Transudate or exudate	Malignant cells	Normal or increased
Tuberculosis peritonitis	Fever, abdominal pain	Exudate	Tubercle bacilli	Normal
Constrictive pericarditis	Inflow stasis	Transudate	——	Increased

phatic obstruction, and portal hypertension. Hypoalbuminemia and secondary hyperaldosteronism are contributory factors. Ascites may be caused by other disorders; that of liver disease must be differentiated from ascites due to tuberculous peritonitis, metastatic malignancy, and constrictive pericarditis. This requires a general medical work-up and a diagnostic paracentesis to obtain fluid for bacteriologic and histologic examination (Box 3).

Severe failure of liver function is characterized by a distinct fetid odor of the breath and by mental clouding which often progresses to coma.[7] The sweetish musty fetor is due to mercaptans,[8] which appear to arise from breakdown of methionine and related substances. Severe liver disease with a poor prognosis is suggested by the presence of intensive fetor in patients not receiving sulfur amino acids in the diet or as a medicament.

BOX 4

HEPATIC COMA

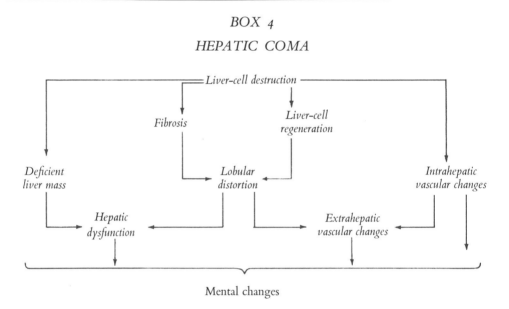

Pathogenesis of hepatic coma

A variety of neuropsychiatric signs and symptoms occur in liver disease. Among them are confusion, lethargy, inappropriate behavior, hypersomnia progressing to inversion of sleep rhythm, momentary disorientation in space, articulatory disturbances, loss of visual acuity, in-co-ordination, "flapping" tremor, apraxia, increased reflexes, and abnormal plantar reflexes. These clinical features are best correlated with electroencephalographic changes and an elevation of blood ammonia (see page 48). Detection of an elevated blood ammonium provides a base line for treatment which consists of the following measures designed to control ammonium intoxication: (1) withholding protein, (2) using broad-spectrum antibiotics to inhibit urea-splitting intestinal bacteria, and (3) supplying glutamic acid or arginine.

Fetor may disappear with improvement in hepatic reserve or upon the administration of antibiotics.

Mental changes are also frequently present and are a grave prognostic sign. Although the etiology of mental changes which are popularly labeled "hepatic encephalopathy" (Figure 7) remains unknown, they are frequently associated with ammonium intoxication and potassium deficiency (Box 4). Pathologic studies show a good correlation between the presence of this condition and hyperplasia of the astrocytes. Electroencephalograms reveal a slowing of the basic rhythm from the normal alpha rhythm; this is similar to alterations seen in uremia and hypoglycemia. The mental changes may be recognized by the occurrence of asterixis,* difficulty in calculation, abnormalities in handwriting, and constructional apraxia.†

Many other signs that are helpful in clinical diagnosis have been noted in patients with liver disease. For example, in alcoholic cirrhosis, parotid swelling (which may become quite prominent) and thickening of the palmar fascia (which occasionally leads to Dupuytren's contracture) are commonly seen and appear to be related to protein malnutrition present in this form of liver disease.

A diffuse brownish skin pigmentation is

*Asterixis, or a flapping tremor, consists in a flexion-extension movement at the wrist elicited by attempted dorsiflexion.

†Constructional apraxia is demonstrable by the inability to reproduce patterns. A convenient test consists in having the patient reproduce a five-point star with matches.

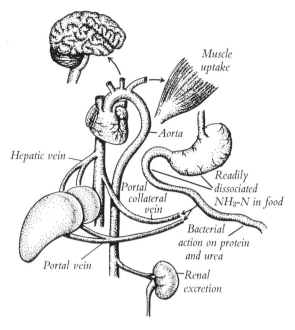

Figure 7. Schematic representation of the mechanism for development of ammonium intoxication.

seen in hemochromatosis, whereas a greenish-yellow ring at the limbus of the cornea (Kayser-Fleischer ring), evidence of lenticular degeneration, or bluish discoloration of the fingernails may represent initial clinical abnormalities in cirrhosis due to Wilson's disease. In terminal liver disease, hemorrhagic tendencies and stigmata of vitamin deficiency, including night blindness, peripheral neuropathy, and papillary atrophy of the tongue, are prominent.

3

Laboratory Recognition of Liver Disease

The foregoing observations have briefly pointed out the more obvious features found in clearly evident liver disease. However, a disorder of the organ frequently exists in the absence of clear-cut signs and symptoms and should be suspected when there is clinical evidence of malnutrition or when a patient has been exposed to known hepatotoxins, received drugs associated with occasional liver injury, been in contact with jaundiced persons, or been given blood transfusions or other parenteral products. Hepatic disease should also be suspected in patients who have unexplained constitutional symptoms, such as fever, weight loss, or malaise. The presence of subclinical alterations of the liver in these instances can be established by means of sensitive biochemical liver function tests and needle biopsy.

More than one hundred different biochemical liver function tests are available, many of them sufficiently sensitive to permit detection of liver disease even in the absence of clinical stigmata. These tests will be discussed in detail later. In general, they are based upon (1) measurement of substances circulating in the blood that depend upon the liver for their production or removal, (2) demonstration of substances in the serum, the levels of which are related to abnormal liver function; (3) study of the plasma disappearance rate of administered dyes and other substances which are removed from the circulation principally by the liver, and (4) measurement of the capacity of the liver to synthesize or produce a given product when an essential precursor is furnished. The major problem in measuring substances produced or removed by the liver is the fact that numerous extrahepatic mechanisms also influence their circulating levels. Such extrahepatic abnormalities have less influence on dye tests and studies designed to evaluate the synthetic capacity of the liver.

Biopsy permits a morphologic diagnosis of liver disease and, consequently, is perhaps the most important of the diagnostic tests. As described subsequently, this technic provides information on the nature, activity, and severity of a hepatic lesion. Tissue obtained by biopsy may also be processed for bacteriologic study or for chemical analysis (Box 5).

Ancillary laboratory studies are essential in patients with established liver disease, since they increase both the diagnostic and the therapeutic perspective. It is desirable to obtain routinely a urinalysis, complete blood count, and chest x-ray. Special laboratory studies should include a hematologic survey in the presence of anemia, cardiovascular studies when there is evidence of heart disease or circulatory congestion, bacteriologic studies when fever or signs of infection are present, gastro-intestinal x-rays in cases of hematemesis or melena, spinal tap and an electroencephalogram when there are mental disturbances, and electrolyte studies in patients with fluid retention or renal dysfunction.

BOX 5

NEEDLE BIOPSY OF LIVER

Needle biopsy of the liver is a relatively simple procedure, although it requires some experience to achieve minimum morbidity. In more than six thousand biopsies performed at the Jersey City Medical Center, only three major complications occurred. Two patients had fatal hemorrhage, and one developed nonfatal bile peritonitis. The low morbidity and mortality in this series are attributed to the fact that only patients with a prothrombin time within two seconds of control values were subjected to biopsy. Furthermore, the biopsy needle was introduced no further than 2 cm. below the surface of the liver. The chief limitation of liver biopsy is related to the size of the sample obtained, which means it is possible to miss localized lesions or to obtain nonrepresentative samples. Although biopsy specimens may be representative of diffuse hepatic parenchymal lesions (such as hepatitis or fatty metamorphosis), they may be misleading in the evaluation of the type and intensity of cirrhosis because of the variability of such lesions throughout the liver. Needles designed for coring, suction, or a combination of these principles are available. Intercostal or subcostal biopsy sites may be used, depending upon the degree of hepatomegaly; peritoneoscopy and photoscans facilitate the detection of localized lesions prior to biopsy.

Continued ➔

Technic with Vim-Silverman needle (coring)   *Technic with Menghini needle (suction)*

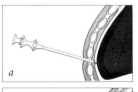 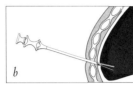
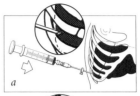 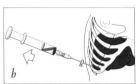
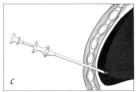 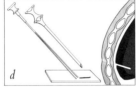
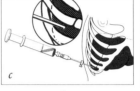 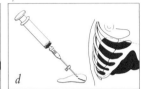

a. *Anesthetize pericapsular tissue.*
   Remove inner stylus.
   Insert outer needle containing inner stylus to just inside hepatic capsule.
b. *Have patient breathe gently or hold breath.*
   Insert bipronged needle to full depth.
c. *Advance outer needle over bipronged needle.*
   Turn outer needle clockwise.
d. *Withdraw both needles simultaneously.*

a. *Anesthetize pericapsular tissue.*
   Preset stopgap.
   Insert needle to hepatic capsule; expel procaine hydrochloride to clear needle.
b. *Pull back on plunger to create vacuum.*
   Have patient breathe gently or hold breath.
c. *Insert needle through hepatic capsule into liver.*
d. *Withdraw needle.*

Indications	Complications	Contraindications
1. *Hepatomegaly of un-determined origin*	1. *Damage to neighboring organs*	1. *Bleeding tendencies*
2. *Confirmation of diagnosis of liver disease*	2. *Bile peritonitis*	2. *Sepsis*
3. *Differential diagnosis of jaundice*	3. *Infection in needle site*	3. *Severe debility*
4. *Therapeutic follow-up of chronic liver disease*	4. *Pain*	4. *Lack of co-operation*
5. *Evaluation of splenomegaly of uncertain origin*	5. *Hemorrhage*	5. *Inability to detect liver dullness*
6. *Fever of unknown origin (granulomas)*	6. *Shock*	

4

Circulatory and Lymphatic Systems

The dynamics of the hepatic circulatory system are influenced by alterations in cardiac output and vascular resistance in peripheral and splanchnic vessels. Congestion associated with heart failure is the most frequent circulatory disturbance which affects the liver. In this condition, stasis of blood is accompanied by hypoxia and leads to ischemic necrosis and fibrosis. The characteristic findings are enlargement and tenderness of the liver in conjunction with altered biochemical function tests; subsequently, in chronic passive congestion, the liver may become small and firm. Marked hepatic congestion is associated with decreased clinical responsiveness to diuretics and digitalis.[9] Similar changes in the liver are noted in shock, when the lower blood pressure results in stasis and accumulation of vasodepressor material.[10]

Liver disease is often accompanied by vascular changes, e.g., an increase in intrasinusoidal and portal pressure, a decrease in estimated hepatic blood flow, opening of collateral vascular channels, and dilatation or blockade of lymph channels. These changes, which are most evident in patients with clinical features of cirrhosis, are responsible for the development of portal hypertension and its complications.

Portal hypertension may be classified as extrahepatic or intrahepatic.[11] The extrahepatic variety consists of conditions which cause portal hypertension by blockade of the portal or hepatic veins, i.e., at the entrance and exit of blood flow through the liver. Intrahepatic portal hypertension is divisible into pre-, para-, and postsinusoidal types, according to the primary location of lesions that interfere with transport of blood through the liver (Table 1).

The liver is occasionally the seat of vascular alterations associated with *occlusion* of such vessels as the hepatic artery, portal vein, hepatic vein, or their branches. There are various causes of vascular occlusion; neoplasm, increased blood coagulability, and polycythe-

Table 1   *PORTAL HYPERTENSION*

Prehepatic	Congenital anomalies Portal vein thrombosis Splenic vein thrombosis Pressure on portal-splenic vein Hepatic artery-portal vein fistula	
Intrahepatic	Laennec's cirrhosis Biliary cirrhosis Postnecrotic cirrhosis Metastatic malignancy Portal fibrosis Wilson's disease Pyelophlebitis Schistosomiasis A-V fistula Congenital hepatic fibrosis Hamartomas	*Presinusoidal*
	Fatty liver Hepatitis Biliary obstruction Postnecrotic cirrhosis Laennec's cirrhosis	*Parasinusoidal*
	Cirrhosis Metastatic malignancy Hepatic vein thrombosis Veno-occlusive disease Constrictive pericarditis	*Postsinusoidal*

Posthepatic	Congestive failure
	Constrictive pericarditis
	Budd-Chiari syndrome:
	    Polycythemia
	    Neoplasm
	    Trauma	

mia are often responsible for the blockade of major blood vessels. Periarteritis nodosa, Wegener's granulomatosis, and aneurysms may involve hepatic arteries, whereas veno-occlusive disease[12] characteristically affects the central veins and their tributaries. The result is different degrees of blood stasis, hypoxia, and ischemic necrosis, depending upon the site of blockade and the availability of collateral circulation.

FUNCTIONAL EVALUATION

Specific study of the vascular system of the liver should be undertaken in patients with chronic liver disease who have symptoms suggestive of portal hypertension or occlusion of a major hepatic blood vessel. Fortunately, the currently available technics provide a number of remarkably diverse approaches for investigating the state of the hepatic circulation. These include (1) estimation of hepatic blood flow and quantitation of collateral circulation, (2) direct or indirect measurement of intrahepatic vascular pressures, (3) radiologic visualization of the hepatic vascular pattern, and (4) morphologic studies of sinusoids, central veins, and portal canals in percutaneous biopsies.

Blood Flow—Much basic and clinical research has been conducted in an effort to devise a simple, accurate bedside method for measuring hepatic blood flow. Attention has been focused primarily on the calculation of blood flow from the disappearance rates of dyes and other substances which theoretically are completely removed from the hepatic blood during each passage through the liver.[13] Although this technic is useful in studies on hepatic physiology, unfortunately it is of no value in liver disease, because removal rates depend upon both blood flow and extraction; with altered liver function, it is not possible to separate these effects.[14] Recently, thermocouples and hydrogen-electrode systems have been incorporated into hepatic vein catheters or inserted directly into the liver to measure hepatic blood flow.[15] Such approaches are in their infancy, but modifications may yield an ideal method for this determination.

At present, the use of the Fick principle (see below) provides the only reliable means of estimating hepatic blood flow. In this procedure, blood flow is calculated by determining the amount of a substance entering (artery) and leaving (hepatic vein) the liver. This method necessitates hepatic vein catheterization. A variety of test agents, including bromsulfalein (BSP),[16] radioiodinated (I[131]) rose bengal,[17] indocyanine green,[18] galactose,[19] and denatured albumin,[20] have been used.

The physical, chemical, and physiologic properties of indocyanine green, in our opinion, make it the best available substance for this purpose. Its only disadvantage is its color, which may interfere with measurement of radioisotopes in the liquid scintillation counter. When measured with this dye, the hepatic blood flow of a normal man is 500 to 800 ml. per minute per square meter of body surface area.[21]

Fick Principle Applied to Hepatic Blood Flow

$$\text{Hepatic blood flow} = \frac{\text{Removal rate*}}{\text{Arterial concentration} - \text{Hepatic vein concentration}} \times \frac{1}{\text{Hematocrit}}$$

*Infusion rate when arterial level is constant.

Because of the significance of both extra-hepatic and intrahepatic collaterals in liver disease with portal hypertension, a number of methods have been developed to identify them and to quantitate their effects. Their visualization is possible by the technics of splenoportography and cineangiography as shown in the discussion of vascular patterns (page 27). The blood flow through collaterals has been investigated by injecting a dye or radioisotope (such as krypton, tritium, or I[131] albumin) into the spleen and determining the time of its appearance in the hepatic venous and systemic circulations.[22]

Pressure Measurements—A knowledge of the degree of portal hypertension would seem to be desirable in all or most patients with chronic liver disease. Portal pressure may be measured directly at the time of operation, or it may be estimated from the pressure in collaterals, such as esophageal varices or hemorrhoidal or abdominal veins. It may also be determined indirectly from the pressure in the splenic pulp or from a catheter "wedged" in an appropriate hepatic vein. (Measurement of esophageal varix pressure is reliable but requires an experienced esophagoscopist.) In the absence of bleeding tendencies, measurement of splenic pulp pressure provides the simplest approach. This may be done at the bedside as described under "Radiologic Visualization of Hepatic Vascular Patterns" (page 27).

In patients with bleeding tendencies or other contraindications to splenic puncture, information on intrahepatic vascular pressure may be obtained by *hepatic vein catheterization.*[23] In this technic, a radiopaque catheter is introduced via a basilic vein and the right atrium (or the femoral vein and inferior vena cava) into an appropriate right or left hepatic vein (Figure 8). When the catheter is introduced, or "wedged," as far as possible into a venule, it prevents the entry of blood into the hepatic vein and produces a static column of blood that transmits the pressure head in the sinusoidal bed to the catheter.

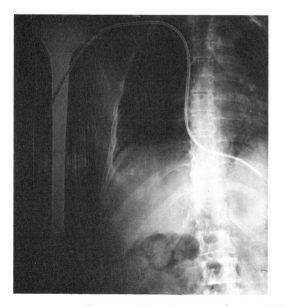 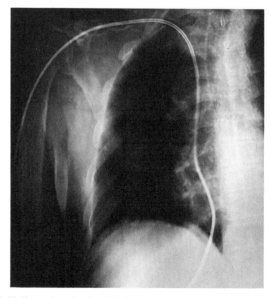

Figure 8. Hepatic vein catheter in left (left) and right (right) hepatic veins.

The intrasinusoidal pressure is a combined effect of portal vein and hepatic artery pressures. In general, the intrasinusoidal pressure (normally 8 to 12 mm. Hg) is raised by an increase in venous or arterial inflow or by obstruction to the outflow. The pressure is lowered by a decrease in entry of blood or by a reduction in sinusoidal resistance.

Hepatic catheterization may be performed in any institution with facilities for cardiovascular catheterization. In addition to measuring pressure, it permits the estimation of hepatic blood flow by the Fick principle, the study of hepatic uptake and release of various substances, and the contrast visualization of the outflow tract of the liver. The procedure is contraindicated in patients with sepsis, debility, and a history of pulmonary embolization and in those who are un-co-operative. At the Jersey City Medical Center, the only complication which developed in more than seven hundred catheterizations was an occasional pyrogenic reaction.

Ideally, combined measurement of intrasplenic pulp pressure and wedged hepatic pressure should be obtained to determine the mechanism of an elevated portal pressure.[10,23] In health, there is a gradual decrease in pressure in the progression from the spleen to the sinusoidal bed of the liver. The splenic pulp pressure is approximately 2 cm. higher than the portal pressure, which is approximately 2 cm. higher than the wedged hepatic vein pressure.

In most instances of portal hypertension, there is a concomitant elevation of both splenic and wedged hepatic pressure (Figure 9). An increased splenic pressure with a normal wedged pressure is characteristic of extrahepatic portal block and of presinusoidal intrahepatic block, such as occurs in schistosomiasis. Normal intrasplenic pressure with an elevated wedged pressure is seen in some pa-

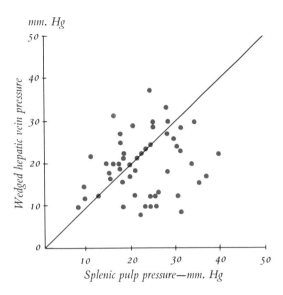

Figure 9. Correlation of wedged hepatic vein pressure and splenic pulp pressure in patients with Laennec's cirrhosis.

tients with extrahepatic collaterals that produce selective decompression of the splenic venous system.

Radiologic Visualization of Hepatic Vascular Patterns—The venous inflow tract of the liver may be visualized by injecting a contrast medium into the spleen (splenoportography). This is a relatively simple technic in which a 4-inch, 19-gauge needle fitted in a polyethylene catheter is introduced at a point over the center of the spleen as estimated by physical examination and fluoroscopy. Fluoroscopy permits one to ascertain that the needle tip is in a venous pool. The needle is withdrawn, but the polyethylene catheter is left in place. A saline manometer is attached for measurement of splenic pulp pressure; 40 ml. of 70 percent sodium acetrizoate are injected into the splenic pulp over a period of two to three seconds, and a serial x-ray or a cineangiogram is taken. This procedure should be undertaken cautiously and is con-

traindicated in the presence of a bleeding tendency, sensitivity to the contrast medium, suspected abscess or tumor of the spleen, renal insufficiency, severe debility, or lack of cooperation. It probably should not be used in patients with jaundice, ascites, or severe anemia. Complications vary with the experience of the operator and selection of patients. Severe pain, uncontrolled hemorrhage, and pyrogenic reactions have been the most common complications at the Jersey City Medical Center. Severe hemorrhage necessitating

splenectomy occurred in 1.5 percent of the patients.

A normal splenoportogram demonstrates contrast medium in the spleen, splenic vein, extrahepatic portal vein, and intrahepatic portal veins. The last are normally long and straight, arborize freely, and approach the liver periphery (Figure 10). Splenoportography has been used clinically to confirm a diagnosis of acquired portal vein thrombosis, to identify cavernomatous transformation, portal vein aplasia, and other congenital le-

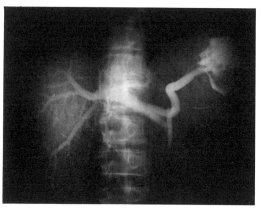

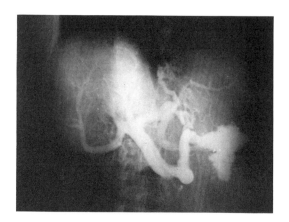

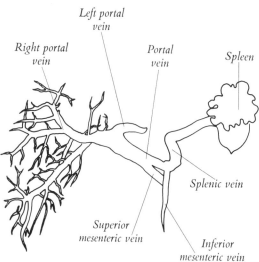

Figure 10. Normal splenoportogram.

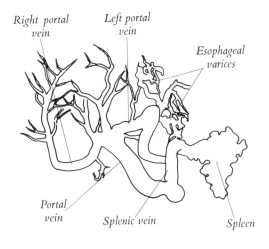

Figure 11. An example of esophageal varices seen on splenoportogram.

sions, to localize hydatid cysts, hemangiomas, and liver abscess, to investigate primary or metastatic carcinoma of the liver, and to evaluate ascites or splenomegaly of undetermined origin. Since it helps to decide the cause of an elevated portal pressure, it is particularly useful in studies of patients with portal hypertension. The procedure aids in identifying esophageal and other collaterals (Figure 11) and in determining the patency of a portacaval shunt postoperatively. Collateral vessels are most often noted in the coronary-esophageal-azygos and the mesenteric venous systems. This technic is desirable in pinpointing the mechanism of gastro-intestinal hemorrhage and encephalopathy in patients with liver disease.

The hepatic venous-outflow tract may be visualized by introducing contrast medium into the liver at the time of hepatic vein catheterization.[10,24] Injecting 50 ml. of an appropriate contrast medium and obtaining x-rays at ten-second intervals usually provide ample visualization. A double-lumen catheter with an inflatable balloon connected to one lumen prevents reflux of the contrast medium and facilitates injection. This technic is of value in determining the patency of the hepatic veins, in locating space-occupying lesions, and in identifying the position of the catheter tip during catheterization (Figure 12).

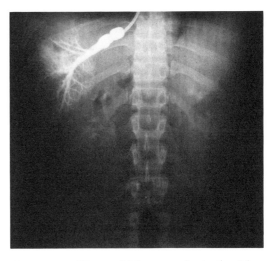

Figure 12. Hepatophlebogram obtained with a special catheter having an inflatable balloon to prevent reflux.

Morphologic Study—Percutaneous biopsies usually permit adequate histologic study of the hepatic vasculature, for at least two or three portal tracts and central veins are present in typical specimens. One may demonstrate such conditions as centrilobular congestion, inflammation, or fibrosis in heart failure,[25] hepatic vein thrombosis (Budd-Chiari syndrome),[26] or veno-occlusive disease.[12] Vasculitis of schistosomiasis, periarteritis nodosa, or Wegener's granulomatosis may first be evident on liver biopsy.

5

Biliary Passages

An important function of the biliary passages is the receipt and excretion of bile pigment. This pigment, bilirubin, which originates in the reticuloendothelial (including Kupffer) cells, is derived largely from the breakdown of aged red cells, from the metabolism of heme in the formation of new red blood cells, and from the turnover of nonhemoglobin heme compounds. This form of bilirubin is unconjugated, is attached to serum albumin, and is lipid soluble. It is transported to the parenchymal liver cells, where microsomal enzymes convert it to water-soluble conjugates of glucuronide (75 percent), sulfate (15 percent), and other substances (10 percent). The now-conjugated bilirubin is excreted through the biliary tract to the intestine, where it is reduced through bacterial action into products such as mesobilirubinogen and stercobilinogen, collectively referred to as "urobilinogen." Urobilinogen is largely excreted in the feces, but some is reabsorbed and reexcreted in the bile or appears in the urine (Figure 13).

FUNCTIONAL EVALUATION

Evaluating the functional state of the biliary network is of immense practical importance, for results of such studies may establish the cause of jaundice and determine whether medical or surgical therapy should be employed. Many tests are available for this. Among the procedures used are (1) direct biochemical analysis of bilirubin in blood, urine, and feces; (2) measurement of blood levels of various nonpigmented substances other than bilirubin which are excreted through the biliary system; (3) evaluation of the disappearance from plasma of dyes that are principally removed from the circulation by the liver and excreted in bile; (4) radiologic visualization of the intrahepatic and extrahepatic biliary radicles; and (5) histologic studies of the biliary network.

Bilirubin Studies—It was Paul Ehrlich who first tested for bilirubin (in the urine) after discovering that the addition of diazotized sulfanilic acid to urine containing bilirubin produced a red color. When applying this test to serum, van den Bergh accidentally discovered that the serum of patients with hemolytic jaundice required the addition of alcohol for the formation of the color, whereas the serum of patients with obstructive jaundice could react "directly," i.e., without the addition of alcohol. This concept of "direct" and "indirect" van den Bergh reactions dominated medical thinking, although clinical correlations were not entirely satisfactory. The

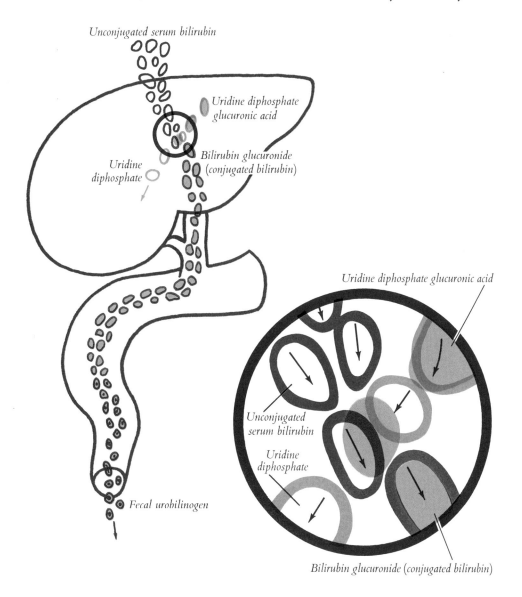

Figure 13. Schematic representation of the conjugation of bilirubin in the liver. The enlarged detail (right) depicts the action of glucuronyl transferase.

BOX 6

MECHANISM OF HYPERBILIRUBINEMIA

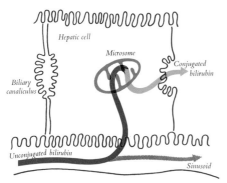

Normal metabolism of bilirubin in liver cell (simplified schema)

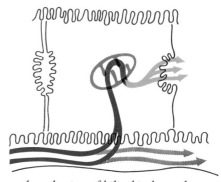

Increased production of bilirubin beyond excretory capacity of the liver (hemolytic jaundice)

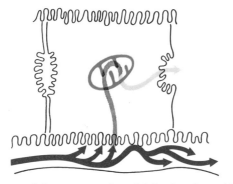

Decreased hepatic uptake of bilirubin (possible mechanism in Gilbert's disease)

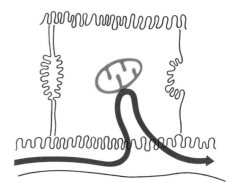

Disturbance in conjugation of bilirubin (e.g., physiologic jaundice of newborn)

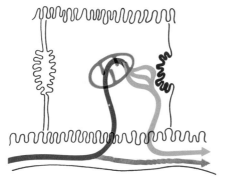

Interference with secretion of conjugated bilirubin into the canaliculi (e.g., Dubin–Johnson syndrome)

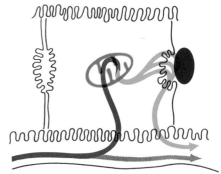

Interference with excretion through intrahepatic and extrahepatic biliary network

puzzle was unraveled almost forty years later when the conjugating function (with glucuronide) of the liver was revealed. Modern hospital laboratories still employ the original technic of measuring conjugated bilirubin in serum by the immediate red color it produces with diazotized sulfanilic acid and of estimating unconjugated bilirubin by the color which develops when alcohol also is added for its stabilizing effect. Nevertheless, the van den Bergh partition is not chemically identical with separation of conjugated and unconjugated bilirubin, since direct-reacting bilirubin is not necessarily conjugated.

A decision as to whether hyperbilirubinemia is of the unconjugated, conjugated, or mixed type represents the first step in determining its mechanism.

Unconjugated hyperbilirubinemia may result from increased production of bilirubin beyond the excretory capacity of the liver (such as occurs in hemolytic states), decreased hepatic uptake of unconjugated bilirubin (as typified by some forms of Gilbert's disease), or lack of conjugation because of a deficiency of enzymes necessary for this process (as seen in the Crigler-Najjar syndrome) (Box 6).

Conjugated hyperbilirubinemia may occur as a result of interference with secretion of bilirubin into the canaliculi or excretion through the intrahepatic or extrahepatic biliary network.

The mixed type—unconjugated and conjugated hyperbilirubinemia—is characteristic of liver-cell disease in which two or more of the above mechanisms may be operative.

A study of bilirubin pigments in the urine provides a simple office method of evaluating the mechanism of hyperbilirubinemia. The normal urine contains 0.5 to 1.4 mg. of urobilinogen per day and no bilirubin. Unconjugated hyperbilirubinemia due to hemolysis or liver-cell injury is characterized by an increase in the urine urobilinogen, whereas, in conjugated hyperbilirubinemia, bilirubin appears in the urine. A variety of methods are available for semiquantitation of urine urobilinogen and bilirubin. These tests are helpful both in recognizing the mechanism of jaundice and in following its course (Box 7).

Similar information may be obtained by a study of fecal bilirubin pigments. The need for collecting twenty-four-hour stool specimens has previously restricted such studies to investigations of the degree of hemolysis in hemolytic jaundice. Normally, 100 to 200 mg. of urobilinogen appear in the feces per twenty-four-hour period; hemolysis usually causes a three-to-fourfold increase in its excretion, and the increment provides a measure of the hemolysis.

Duodenal drainage, once widely used in study of the jaundiced patient, has again become popular and may be extremely useful in differential diagnosis. Microscopic examination of a suitable aspirate often provides evidence of malignant cells or calculi. For this purpose, assessment of the bile content of the aspirate is particularly helpful during early phases of jaundice. In complete extrahepatic biliary obstruction, there is usually no bilirubin in the fasting state or following intravenous cholecystokinin. In contrast, cholecystokinin usually evokes a release of bile in *incomplete* intrahepatic or extrahepatic biliary obstruction. Occasionally, confusion may arise since, during the initial phases of *complete* intrahepatic or extrahepatic biliary obstruction (above the entrance of the gall bladder), cholecystokinin may also evoke a release of some bile.

Other Excretory Products—Lesions which obstruct bile outflow are accompanied by an increase in the serum concentration of cholesterol and in activities of such enzymes as aminoleucine peptidase, alkaline phosphatase, and transaminase. Measurement of these substances in the serum may be helpful in confirming a diagnosis of biliary obstruction, although they may be increased because of overproduction or a metabolic defect. When interpreting results, one should be aware of the influence of nonhepatic processes on their circulatory levels. Of these substances, the serum *alkaline phosphatase* is most consistently helpful in assessing hepatic excretory function (see Figure 21, page 54). Several different chemical procedures are available for its determination. The increase in alkaline phos-

---

BOX 7

MEASUREMENT OF URINE UROBILINOGEN

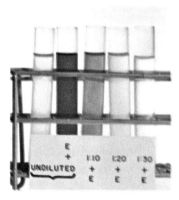

Normal urine   *Increased urobilinogen*

Addition of 0.5 ml. of Ehrlich's aldehyde reagent (paradimethylaminobenzaldehyde) (E) produces a red color which is present to a dilution of 1:20.

Addition of 0.5 ml. of Ehrlich's aldehyde (E) produces a red color which is present beyond a dilution of 1:20.

A study of urine bilirubin pigments represents the first and most readily available approach to the differential diagnosis of jaundice. In measuring urine urobilinogen, it is essential to have a freshly voided urine specimen from a patient not receiving antibiotics. Stagnation is associated with oxidation of urine urobilinogen to urobilin, and antibiotics suppress bacteria that are necessary for the conversion of bilirubin to urobilinogen in the intestines. Diarrhea may also interfere with urobilinogen production. When bilirubin is present in the urine, it should be removed by adding 10 percent barium chloride to 5 ml. of urine and filtering it before testing for urobilinogen.

Urine bilirubin and urobilinogen should be measured simultaneously. Commercial tablets are available for semiquantitative analysis of urine bilirubin. The semiquantitative Wallace-Diamond method or quantitative methods may be used for urobilinogen.

phatase due to biliary obstruction must be differentiated from that seen in bone disease. Clinical features, bone x-rays, and electrophoretic demonstration of alkaline phosphatase in the alpha-globulin (liver) rather than the beta-globulin (bone) fraction of plasma proteins usually make this possible.[27]

Dyes—Dyes are widely used to assess hepatic excretory function. However, they are of limited value in determining the functional status of the biliary network, for their removal from the plasma also depends upon liver-cell function. Maximum information is obtained by a serial study of plasma dye levels, particular attention being given to the excretory phase, which usually begins thirty to forty minutes after administration of the dye. In the absence of icterus, *bromsulfalein* (BSP) is the most useful of currently available dyes in detecting early lesions of the biliary tract. Norethandrolone (Nilevar®), an anabolic steroid, and its analogues regularly cause an abnormal plasma removal of BSP which can be correlated with the morphologic changes induced in the canaliculi by these drugs.[28]

We have found *indocyanine green* to be the safest and most useful dye in assessing excretory function in the presence of icterus. It is of particular value in studies of patients with unconjugated hyperbilirubinemia (in which its removal kinetics are normal) and in familial conjugated hyperbilirubinemia (in which its initial removal is within normal limits but its excretory phase is abnormal). Radioiodinated (I[131]) *rose bengal* has proved to be of greatest value in hyperbilirubinemia due to biliary obstruction. It does not permit differentiation between intrahepatic and extrahepatic obstruction, but it has the advantage of not requiring blood samples from infants with suspected biliary obstruction (Box 8).[29]

Cholecystography and Cholangiography— The diagnostic value of radiologic studies of the biliary network is well established. Available technics include oral, intravenous, operative, and percutaneous cholangiography. When using any of these methods, one must be constantly aware of the potential hypersensitivity to gall-bladder dyes and the occasional occurrence of anaphylactoid reactions, icterus,[30] or renal insufficiency.[31]

Oral cholecystography (in which six or twelve tablets of iodopanoic acid or other contrast media are used) is the simplest of these procedures. There is usually nonvisualization of the gall bladder in jaundice due to acquired liver-cell dysfunction, and, in most instances, cholecystography is neither helpful nor desirable. In cirrhosis, the ability of the gall bladder to be visualized on x-ray is directly related to the severity of the liver disease. In patients with cirrhosis without evidence of hepatic failure, a normal response occurs. In patients with cirrhosis accompanied by jaundice, ascites, or hepatic fetor, nonvisualization is characteristic. In such cases, improvement in hepatic reserve may be followed by restoration of the capacity of the gall bladder to be visualized.

In constitutional hyperbilirubinemia and in the Crigler-Najjar syndrome, the gall bladder is normally visualized; it is not, however, in the Dubin-Johnson syndrome, and this aids in the differential diagnosis. Because of the high incidence of cholelithiasis in patients over fifty years of age, cholecystography may be of value in subjects with liver disease accompanied by intermittent hyperbilirubinemia or symptoms compatible with gallstones. Normal visualization is to be expected in metastatic liver disease and hepatic congestion without jaundice, as well as in acute virus hepatitis when the serum bilirubin is less than 4 mg. per 100 ml.

BOX 8

DYE EXTRACTION BY THE LIVER

Bromsulfalein (BSP)   Indocyanine green (ICG)   Rose bengal

Three dyes, bromsulfalein (BSP), indocyanine green (ICG), and radioiodinated rose bengal, have been used principally to assess the functional state of the liver. The physical and chemical properties of these dyes differ considerably. BSP and rose bengal are anionic phthalein dyes, whereas ICG is a tricarbo-cyanine dye.

BSP is bound to plasma protein following its intravenous administration; 70 to 80 percent is removed from the bloodstream by the liver, and the rest is removed by extrahepatic mechanisms. BSP secreted into the bile and urine may be separated into "free" dye and at least three amino acid conjugates—glutamic acid, glycine, and cystine. BSP has the disadvantage of being extremely irritating when injected subcutaneously and can produce allergic or anaphylactoid reactions (e.g., nausea, vomiting, skin eruptions, shock, or, rarely, death).

The physical properties of ICG (originally introduced for estimation of cardiac output by the indicator dilution technic) contrast sharply with those described for BSP. Over 95 percent of the administered ICG can be recovered from bile; it is not excreted as a conjugate, and it does not undergo an extrahepatic circulation. It is nonirritating when introduced subcutaneously, and no untoward effect has been noted from its repeated injection. The physical characteristics of ICG make it possible to measure its arterial level by dichromatic ear densitometry. This principle is widely used in estimating cardiac output. Studies in the Jersey City Medical Center indicate that the Waters dichromatic ear densitometer may be utilized to determine the level of ICG during a constant infusion[21] or to evaluate its hepatic uptake after a single injection. This approach constitutes a major advancement in the evaluation of hepatic function in chronic liver disease, since it provides a simpler method for serial study of the percentage disappearance rate and half-life of ICG.

Rose bengal has a physiologic behavior similar to that of ICG; substitution of a gamma-emitting isotope, I^{131}, for the iodine in the rose bengal molecule permits studies of dye uptake, storage, and excretion by means of external scintillation counting. Removal of these dyes from the plasma is dependent upon the status of both the liver cell, which determines their uptake and storage, and the biliary tract, which governs their excretion.

Intravenous cholangiography is particularly helpful in cholecystectomized patients who have evidence of biliary tract dysfunction and in subjects in whom an oral gall-bladder dye is poorly tolerated. Cholangiography is indispensable in differentiating between intrahepatic and extrahepatic biliary obstruction. Percutaneous hepatic cholangiography (in which a contrast medium is injected directly into a bile duct—reached by blind puncture with aspiration) has been recommended for this purpose since intravenous cholangiography is usually not successful. This technic has been found quite useful in recognizing extrahepatic biliary obstruction which, unlike the intrahepatic obstruction, is usually associated with dilatation of the major biliary radicles. Since the major complication of percutaneous cholangiography is bile peritonitis, it should be performed by or in co-operation with a surgeon prepared for immediate surgical intervention. Abdominal exploration with operative T-tube cholangiography (Figure 14) and liver biopsy is desirable when there is a lack of experience with percutaneous cholangiography and in cases of persistent biliary obstruction in which this procedure does not reveal dilated ducts.

Histologic Studies—The chief value of percutaneous liver biopsy in the jaundiced patient is in establishing the location and nature of intrahepatic lesions. Morphologic studies permit a definite demonstration of parenchymal-cell disturbances, such as hepatitis, fatty liver, cirrhosis, or infiltrative lesions, which may cause secondary excretory dysfunction. A normal histologic picture is present in unconjugated hyperbilirubinemia resulting from Gilbert's disease or the Crigler-Najjar syndrome; also, the hepatic structure is not altered in many instances of hemolytic jaundice. Hemolysis associated with sickle-cell

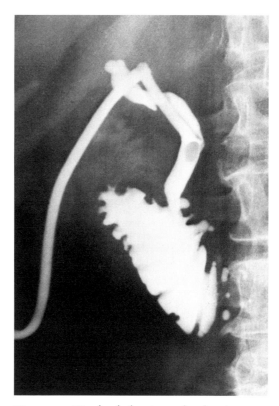

Figure 14. T-tube cholangiography showing stone in common duct.

crises is an exception in that red-cell phagocytosis by Kupffer cells and dilatation with puddling of red cells in sinusoids are characteristic. When the location of the obstruction is not known in patients with conjugated hyperbilirubinemia, surgical intervention is desirable to differentiate intrahepatic cholestasis from extrahepatic biliary obstruction. Biopsy and cholangiographic studies can then be performed if an extrahepatic lesion is not demonstrable. Careful conventional microscopic study by an experienced pathologist may permit discovery of primary changes in the microvilli of the bile canaliculi, delineate inflammation, proliferation, or destruction of bile ductules, or reveal inflammation and injury of bile ducts.

6

Reticuloendothelial Cells

The "reticuloendothelial" system was originally defined as a combination of endothelial cells with reticulum cells. The term is now used in a variety of ways. Some restrict it to phagocytic cells, whereas others include a variety of other mesenchymal cells. Fine structural examination has demonstrated the presence of at least five different types of "RE," or sinusoidal, cells—endothelial, phagocytic, gamma-globulin-synthesizing, fiber-forming, and hematic cells.[32] Attention has been centered chiefly on the stellate phagocytic sinusoidal (Kupffer) cells, which function primarily as macrophages. These cells phagocytize foreign and endogenous substances and sequester red cells released by intravascular hemolysis; this capacity depends upon particle size and coating of material to be engulfed. The immunocytic variety of sinusoidal cells produce antibodies which may contribute to resistance to infection or lead to hypersensitivity states.

The importance of the hepatic "RE," or sinusoidal, cells in evaluating the over-all state of liver function is related to the fact that (1) a variety of substances, such as iron, vitamin A, and lipids, are stored in hepatic Kupffer cells, and such storage may interfere with the cells' essential phagocytic function; and (2) any nonfatal hepatic injury produces pro-liferation of mesenchymal and ductular cells, which may lead to observed clinical and laboratory abnormalities. It has been shown that proliferation of the immunocytic variety of sinusoidal cells is accompanied by an elevated serum globulin. Some investigators believe that an increase in endothelial and fiber-forming sinusoidal cells contributes to portal hypertension, ischemia, and further hepatic damage.[33]

FUNCTIONAL EVALUATION

The sinusoidal cells of the liver may be best evaluated through histologic studies. Their phagocytic capacity may be investigated by a study of the disappearance rate of various substances which they selectively remove from the circulation. Their immunocytic activity may be roughly assessed by measurement of serum gamma globulin and more precisely by immunocytochemical studies. Ordinary light microscopy shows that the stellate phagocytic sinusoidal (Kupffer) cells accumulate iron in a variety of conditions and store lipids in Gaucher's and in Niemann-Pick's disease. The availability of tritium-labeled thymidine, a precursor of deoxyribonucleic acid (DNA), has permitted the in-vitro investigation of nucleic acid synthesis in sinusoidal (reticuloendothelial) cells from percutaneous biopsy specimens of the human liver (Box 9).

Human liver tissue, obtained by percutaneous biopsy, is incubated in vitro with this radioisotope. Results indicate that most cases of liver damage in man are characterized by proliferation of mesenchymal cells. By this technic, the normal ratio of labeled mesenchymal cells to liver cells is 4:1. In acute liver injury, this ratio may increase up to 10:1 owing to mesenchymal-cell proliferation. It may decrease to 1:1 in the recovery phases of liver injury because of a relatively greater increase in labeled liver cells. The turnover of mesenchymal cells is best correlated with the presence of active necrosis; however, despite necrosis, cell turnover is diminished or absent when there is a deficiency of enzymes or substrates necessary for DNA or ribonucleic acid (RNA) synthesis, when deoxyribonuclease or other inhibitors are present, or when there is irreversible injury to the template of DNA.

The disappearance from the circulation of colloidal gold,[34] colloidal carbon, and I^{131}-labeled denatured albumin[35] has been used to estimate phagocytic function of sinusoidal

---

BOX 9

DNA SYNTHESIS IN PERCUTANEOUS LIVER BIOPSIES

An autoradiographic technic employing tritium-labeled thymidine may be used to assess DNA synthesis in vitro in percutaneous liver biopsies from man. This technic permits the objective assessment of the regenerative response in patients with liver disease. The nutritional status and specific therapeutic agents have a significant effect on labeling patterns. Acute nonfatal liver injury primarily causes an increase in proliferation of mesenchymal cells and lesser degrees of proliferation of the ductular and liver cells. This procedure may be helpful in determining the prognosis of liver disease in an individual patient and in the objective evaluation of the effectiveness of various forms of therapy.

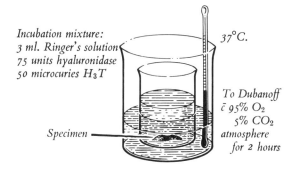

Incubation mixture:
3 ml. Ringer's solution
75 units hyaluronidase
50 microcuries H_3T

37°C.

To Dubanoff
c̄ 95% O_2
5% CO_2
atmosphere
for 2 hours

Specimen

Liver biopsies are obtained with the Vim–Silverman needle and split longitudinally. One half is immediately immersed in a solution containing tritiated thymidine and hyaluronidase. After incubation for one and one-half hours, the tissue is removed and standard technics are used to prepare autoradiographs.

Continued →

cells; however, none of these substances has been of value in clinical practice. Recently, a specially prepared lipid emulsion, which is removed from the vascular system by RE cells, has been employed for this purpose. The "half-time" was significantly decreased in patients with bacterial infections.[36]

Hyperplasia of the immunocytic variety of hepatic sinusoidal cells is associated with a marked increase in serum gamma globulin. In fact, there is a good correlation between the proliferation of such cells and elevation of gamma globulin. Examination of the electrophoretic protein patterns permits the detection of these marked increases in globulin, and deviations in the cephalin flocculation or the thymol turbidity test provide a clinical clue to the abnormality. Immunocytochemical data have been obtained by treating frozen human biopsy specimens with rabbit anti-human gamma globulins and examining them under the fluorescent microscope.[37]

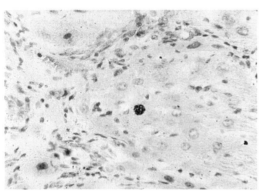

A single labeled liver cell in autoradiograph of biopsy specimen of inactive cirrhosis. The heavy labeled cell represents the one which has taken up tritiated thymidine. (450x)

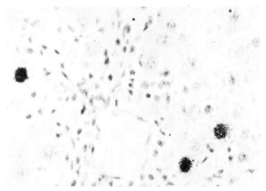

Multiple labeled liver cells in autoradiograph of biopsy specimen of active virus hepatitis. (450x)

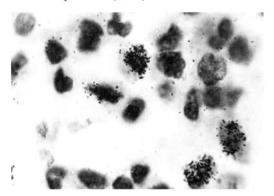

Multiple labeled neoplastic liver cells in autoradiograph of biopsy specimen of hepatoma. (900x)

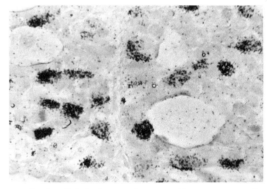

Multiple labeled neoplastic cells in autoradiograph of biopsy specimen of metastatic adenocarcinoma to liver. (900x)

7

Parenchymal Cells

The multiple functions of the liver cell make it more difficult to determine its "status" than that of any other cell in the body. Ideally, perhaps, one should assess the "function" of the hepatic cell by studying the status of its component parts. These "organelles" may be visualized directly by combined light and electron microscopy, or they may be separated for analysis by ultracentrifugation. Such studies have greatly increased our understanding of the liver cell and emphasize the integrated function of all of its elements.

The normal human liver cell contains a nucleus, mitochondria, lysosomes, and endoplasmic reticula, each of which has discrete functions (Figure 15).

Morphologic studies of the *nucleus* indicate that it has a double membrane containing pores which permit exchange of material with cell cytoplasm. It normally contains 46 chromosomes but often has 92, 138, or more (polyploidy).

Most interest has been concentrated on the approximately 400 *mitochondria*, the "power plants" of the cell, since they conduct the primary energy transformations of the cells. They contain the Krebs citric acid cycle enzymes in the matrix and enzymes governing electron transport and oxidative phosphorylation in their membrane covering. Mitochondria may be identified by the presence of a double membrane, the inner one being invaginated to form cristae.

The *reticulum* consists of lamellae profiles which are designated as "rough" and "smooth" reticula. The rough reticulum represents ribosomes, which are the site of protein synthesis. Endoplasmic reticulum associated with ribosomes is responsible for synthesis of circulating proteins, whereas cellular proteins are produced in the ribosome-free reticulum. The smooth reticulum is the site of drug detoxification and activity of enzymes necessary for conjugation of bilirubin and formation of glycogen (Figures 15a and 15b).

Lysosomes were the last of these subcellular organelles to be described. They are denser and slightly smaller bodies than mitochondria and serve intracellular digestion, storage, and secretion. They contain hydrolytic enzymes, including ribonuclease, deoxyribonuclease, phosphatases, cathepsins, glycosidases, and sulfatases. The fascinating studies of de Duve suggest that these enzymes dissolve the substances ingested by the cell and, under certain circumstances, can dissolve the cell itself.

Liver-cell damage (resulting from a host of causes, including nutritional deficiency, infectious agents, hepatotoxins, circulatory congestion, or biliary obstruction) is characterized by an alteration of subcellular structures.

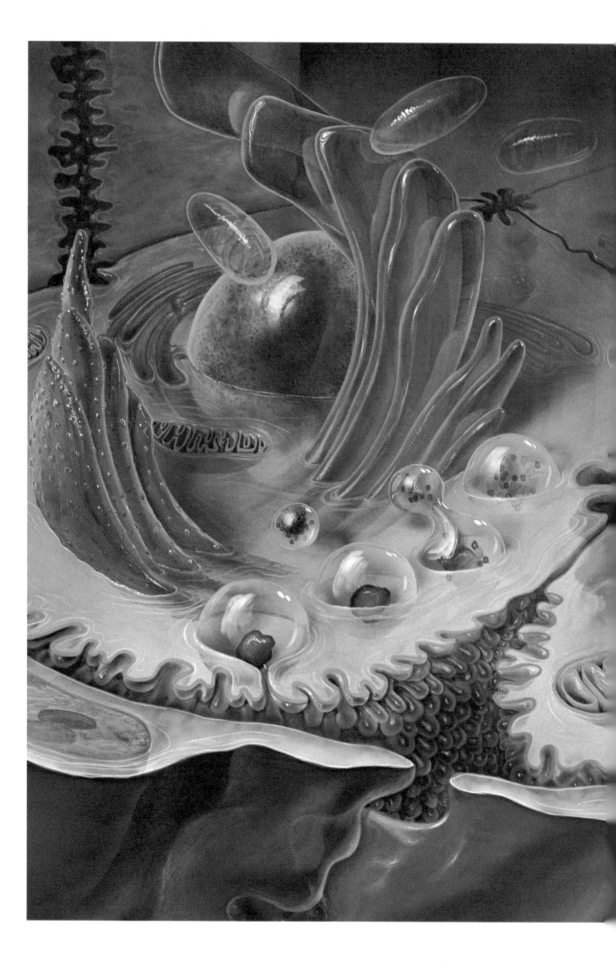

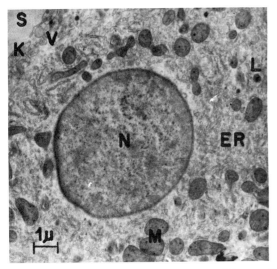

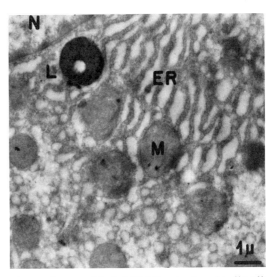

Figure 15a. Electron microscope view of liver cell. The nucleus is labeled "N," mitochondria "M," lysosomes "L," endoplasmic reticula "ER," sinusoid "S," Kupffer cell "K" lining the sinusoid, and microvilli "V" projecting into the space of Disse.

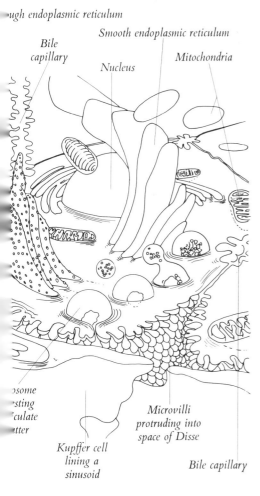

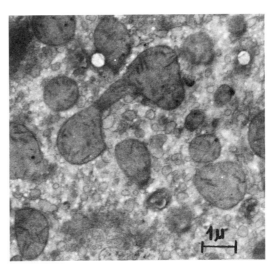

Figure 15b. Normal mitochondria (above) compared with swollen and degenerated mitochondria (below).

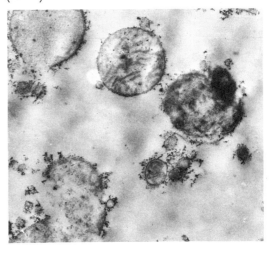

ugh endoplasmic reticulum

Bile
capillary

Smooth endoplasmic reticulum

Nucleus

Mitochondria

osome
sting
culate
tter

Kupffer cell
lining a
sinusoid

Microvilli
protruding into
space of Disse

Bile capillary

ure 15. Schematic representation of the struc-
of a hepatic cell.

This may be reflected by a change in their size or staining qualities and/or by evidence of necrosis on light microscopy. Such damage evokes a regenerative reaction which varies in intensity depending upon the capacity of the undamaged cells to synthesize nucleic acids and other cellular elements.

In man, reproduction of liver cells appears to occur at a slower rate than that of other cellular elements of the liver.[38] New liver cells may imitate embryonal and neonatal development and appear in plates two to three cells thick rather than in the unicellular cords characteristic of the normal liver. A combination of fibrogenesis, bile-duct proliferation, and nodular regeneration of liver cells causes

---

BOX 10

PROTEIN PATTERNS IN LIVER DISEASE

| Normal serum protein pattern | Active postnecrotic cirrhosis *(decreased albumin and increased beta and gamma globulin)* | Active primary biliary cirrhosis *(decreased albumin and increased beta globulin)* |

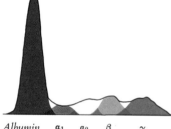 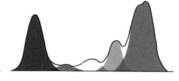 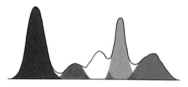

Albumin   α₁   α₂   β   γ

The technic of paper electrophoresis permits the ready identification of abnormalities in serum protein fractions. The total serum protein concentration may be measured by a Kjeldahl nitrogen method. By means of immunoelectrophoretic analysis, one may identify the components of various electrophoretically separated fractions. Alpha-1 globulin contains glycoprotein, alpha lipoprotein, and many enzymes; alpha-2 globulin contains hemoglobin-binding glycoprotein (or haptoglobin), copper-binding protein (or ceruloplasmin), alpha-2 lipoprotein, and alpha-2 microglobulin. Iron-binding globulin (or transferrin), heme-binding protein (or hemopexin), and the complement fraction beta lipoprotein are present in beta globulin.

Gamma globulins (the immune globulins) consist of the fractions gamma-2, gamma-1A, and gamma-1M. Normal serum contains 800 to 1,100 mg. per 100 ml. of gamma-2 globulin, which has a molecular weight of approximately 170,000 and a sedimentation constant of 7 Svedberg (S) units and contains natural antibodies, anti-O antibodies, and isoagglutinins. Serum also contains 50 to 100 mg. per 100 ml. of gamma-1A globulin, which is similar in molecular weight and sedimentation constant to gamma-2 globulin and appears to contain skin-sensitizing antibodies. In addition, normal serum contains 50 to 70 mg. of gamma-1M globulin, which has a molecular weight of approximately 1,000,000, has a sedimentation constant of 19S, and contains antitoxins, anti-H antibodies, and antibodies to bacteria and viruses.

the lobular distortion that is characteristic of cirrhosis.

FUNCTIONAL EVALUATION

In clinical practice, the functional status of the parenchymal cells may be evaluated by (1) measuring the serum concentration of substances produced by the liver cell; (2) determining the serum content of substances whose level is changed by liver-cell damage; (3) evaluating the serum activity levels of enzymes released from the liver cell as a result of injury; (4) determining the ability of the liver to perform a metabolic task, such as acceptance and secretion of dyes, conjugation, or detoxification; (5) measuring enzyme and substrate content of liver tissue; and (6) microscopic study of the liver cell and its subcellular organelles.

Serum Concentration of Certain Substances — The liver cell is responsible for the synthesis of serum albumin, alpha and beta globulin, plasma enzymes, glycoproteins, and lipoproteins. It is also a major site of plasma protein catabolism. The serum concentrations of a large number of substances produced by the liver have been measured in the assessment of liver-cell function. Probably the most readily performed studies in the clinical laboratory concern plasma proteins. Hepatic disease is often characterized by alterations in plasma protein fractions, which may be detected by electrophoresis (Box 10).

Plasma of patients with liver disease also frequently exhibits a deficiency of a variety of constituents present in healthy subjects. The most prominent deficiency leading to observed clinical abnormalities is that of protein factors concerned with clotting — proaccelerin, fibrinogen, and vitamin-K-dependent clotting factors. Bleeding tendencies in liver disease occur as a result of a deficiency of

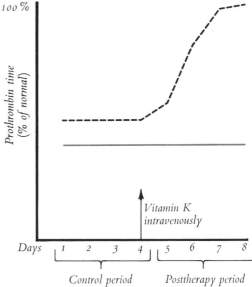

——— Patient with severe liver disease and hypoprothrombinemia due to inability to produce prothrombin. Note: Administration of vitamin K had no effect on hypoprothrombinemia.

- - - - Patient with extrahepatic biliary obstruction and hypoprothrombinemia due to inability to absorb vitamin K. Note: Vitamin K caused rapid increase of low prothrombin to normal range.

Figure 16. Use of vitamin K in the clinical differential diagnosis of jaundice associated with hypoprothrombinemia.

these and other plasma clotting factors. Platelet abnormalities, the presence of circulating anticoagulants, and increased plasma fibrinolysis may also be contributory.[39] Several substances (Christmas factor, factor VII, Stuart factor, and prothrombin) are frequently deficient in patients with liver disease.

The one-stage prothrombin time[40] performed before and after administration of vitamin K permits detection of these abnormalities and is useful in differentiating deficiencies caused by abnormal vitamin K absorption from those due to liver-cell dysfunction (Figure 16). Responsiveness of an abnormal prothrombin time to vitamin **K** has been widely used as a method to distinguish between obstructive and hepatocellular jaundice. Biliary obstruction interferes with absorption of this vitamin; when it is administered parenterally, the prothrombin returns to normal. In contrast, in jaundice and hypoprothrombinemia due to liver-cell damage, vitamin K has little or no effect on the prothrombin time.

Serum Constituents Changed in Liver Damage—Empirical tests based upon some qualitative or quantitative physicochemical alterations in serum proteins have been widely used to detect liver disease and follow its course. When properly performed, they provide insight into the activity of hepatic lesions and are useful in the differential diagnosis of jaundice. The cephalin flocculation and thymol turbidity tests are the most commonly used of this group in the hospital laboratory. The *cephalin flocculation* may be abnormal because of a change in the concentration of a stabilizing fraction relative to a given amount of gamma globulin[41] or because of a reaction to a special fraction of gamma globulin.[42] The *thymol turbidity* test is positive because of a relative increase in gamma globulin and beta lipoprotein.[43]

Enzyme Release—Enzymes and substrates which are involved in intermediary metabolism and stored in high concentration in the

Table 2

PLASMA ENZYMES OF VALUE IN DIAGNOSIS OF LIVER DISEASE

Recognition of Liver-Cell Damage

1. Transaminases Serum glutamic oxalacetic transaminase (SGOT) Serum glutamic pyruvic transaminase (SGPT)	Of principal value in recognition and follow-up of hepatitis. Increased values must be differentiated from those caused by extrahepatic lesions.
2. Dehydrogenases Lactic acid dehydrogenase Isocitric acid dehydrogenase	Of principal value in recognizing hepatitis and differentiating it from other lesions, such as myocardial infarction.

Recognition of Biliary Obstruction

1. Alkaline phosphatase	May be increased in infiltrative lesions of liver or in bone disease.
2. Leucine aminopeptidase	Of major value in complete biliary obstruction.

Infiltrative Lesions of the Liver

1. Alkaline phosphatase	Abnormal in 40 percent of advanced lesions.
2. Isocitric acid dehydrogenase	Abnormal in 20 to 30 percent of advanced lesions.

liver cell are often released when there is acute hepatic-cell damage. The resulting increase in serum concentration of released enzymes provides a valuable diagnostic clue to the presence and activity of a lesion involving the liver cell (Table 2).

The serum glutamic oxalacetic transaminase (SGOT) and serum glutamic pyruvic *transaminase* (SGPT) determinations are the most sensitive of the available enzyme tests

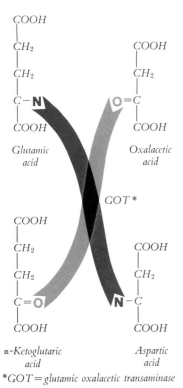

COOH
|
CH₂
|
CH₂
|
C — N
|
COOH

Glutamic acid

COOH
|
CH₂
|
O = C
|
COOH

Oxalacetic acid

GOT *

COOH
|
CH₂
|
CH₂
|
C = O
|
COOH

α-Ketoglutaric acid

COOH
|
CH₂
|
N — C
|
COOH

Aspartic acid

GOT = glutamic oxalacetic transaminase

*Figure 17. Transfer of an amino group from an amino acid to an **α**-keto acid—a function of a transaminase.*

in liver disease (Figure 17). Myocardial infarction, circulatory congestion, muscle injury, central-nervous-system diseases, postoperative states, and other nonhepatic conditions in which the enzymes are increased must be excluded in relating observed abnormalities to

hepatic injury. Serum transaminase determinations are of the greatest value in virus hepatitis, in which they are significantly increased and then slowly return to normal with healing. Alcoholics with jaundice, leukocytosis, fever, and marked hyaline necrosis frequently have a normal serum and low liver pyruvic transaminase. Recent studies indicate that such persons also have a vitamin B_6 deficiency and that the low content of pyruvic transaminase in the liver may be due to a lack of vitamin B_6 or its apoenzyme.[44]

The inability to ascribe increases of transaminases to liver injury per se may be partly resolved by the concomitant measurement of the enzyme *lactic dehydrogenase*. It has been shown that lactic dehydrogenase exists in five electrophoretically distinct molecular varieties and that the proportion of lactic dehydrogenase isoenzymes is specific for each tissue. Consequently, serum lactic dehydrogenase released from the liver has less electrophoretic mobility than that released from the heart and, unlike cardiac lactic dehydrogenase, is not inhibited by sulfite.[45] The ability to separate lactic dehydrogenase according to its tissue origin may, therefore, aid in determining whether the enzymes have been released from liver cells.

Measurement of serum vitamin B_{12} is also valuable, since this vitamin is not affected by most of the nonhepatic conditions which cause elevation of transaminase.[46] The availability of specific and sensitive microbiologic technics for measuring it permits its use as a clinical diagnostic aid (Figure 18). In hepatic-cell necrosis, there is a release of vitamin B_{12} from the liver into the serum; the serum, which normally contains about 100 to 900 μμg. of vitamin B_{12} per ml. (as assayed with *Ochromonas malhamensis*), may exhibit levels as high as 2,000 to 3,000 μμg. per ml. The serum vitamin B_{12} level remains elevated

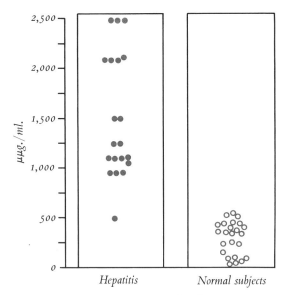

Figure 18. Serum vitamin B$_{12}$ levels in acute virus hepatitis.

with continuing liver injury and returns to normal when active liver-cell necrosis subsides. Increases of vitamin B$_{12}$ may not occur in malnourished subjects depleted of the vitamin; therefore, results of this test may be misleading in liver disease in the alcoholic patient.

Metabolic Performance—A quantitative measurement of the ability of the liver to metabolize specific endogenous or exogenous substances is an excellent method for assessing the functional capacity of the liver cell. Any of the large number of metabolic tasks which the liver cell performs may be used for this purpose. However, only those which can be performed simply in the clinical laboratory are useful. Four tests have been found to be acceptable for this purpose—determination of blood ammonia, serum cholesterol ester, galactose tolerance, and hippuric acid synthesis. The simplest and most widely used of this group is the measurement of *blood ammonia*.

Assessment of the role of the liver in ammonia fixation provides a good index to the functional state of the liver cell. It has three mechanisms for ammonia fixation: synthesis of the carbamyl phosphate precursor of urea and pyrimidines, synthesis of glutamine, and reductive reamination of *a*-ketoglutaric acid. An elevated fasting arterial ammonia is often noted with severe liver disease, and hyperammoniemia shows a good, although not perfect, correlation with the mental state. Administration of either a 60-Gm.-protein test meal or 2 Gm. of ammonium chloride causes no significant rise in the blood ammonia over a four-hour period in the normal subject or in patients with mild liver disease. In contrast, a significant rise in blood ammonia occurs with severe liver disease or development of collaterals (Figure 19).[47]

Over 60 percent of the serum *cholesterol* is normally present in the form of an ester of polyunsaturated fatty acids. Cholesterol-esterifying activity depends on the presence of a transferase enzyme.[48] Liver-cell damage is characterized by a reduction in the absolute amount of cholesterol esters.

The intravenous *galactose tolerance* test, which measures the capacity of the liver cell to convert galactose to glucose, is no longer used because of the need for measuring both circulating galactose and glucose. It is often difficult to interpret the simpler oral test, since its results also depend upon intestinal and renal function.

The intravenous *hippuric acid synthesis* test is designed to evaluate the ability of the liver cell to convert benzoic acid into hippuric acid. It, also, is only infrequently used at present because of the availability of simpler laboratory procedures.

Tissue Levels—Tissue levels of a large number of substances have been measured in specimens of liver obtained from man. These procedures are usually tedious and have been used principally for research. Although it has been demonstrated that there may not be any relationship between tissue content and circulating products, the ability to determine the chemical composition of subcellular fractions of the liver makes this an important area for future work.

A variety of enzymes and substrates have been measured in the human liver to date; these include glycogen, potassium, folic acid, vitamin B$_{12}$, pyridoxine, adenosine triphosphate, pyridine nucleotides, alcohol dehydrogenase, and transaminases. The derived values have been expressed in relation to dry or wet weight, nitrogen content, or nucleic acid content of the liver specimen. Such observations may be of great practical importance in the management of liver disease. For example, it has been shown that the diseased liver is frequently depleted of folic acid, vita-

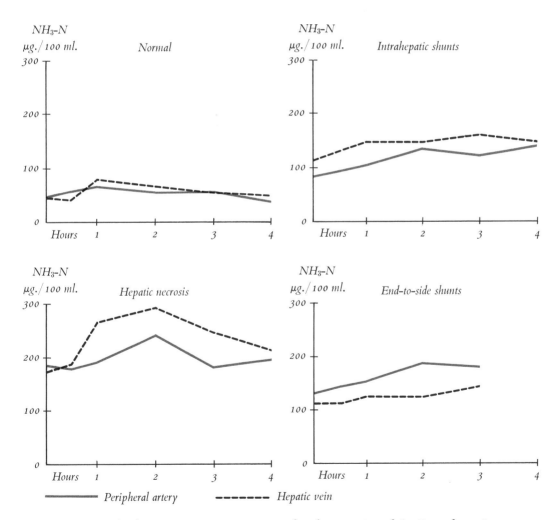

Figure 19. Blood ammonia nitrogen patterns after the ingestion of 60 Gm. of protein.

min B$_{12}$, pyridoxine, or adenosine triphosphate, all of which are essential for its regeneration. Similarly, decreased tolerance for alcoholic beverages and morphine in patients with liver disease has been related to encountered reduction in alcohol dehydrogenase and transferase respectively.

Morphology—Microscopic study of the liver cell still provides the best method for assessing its functional state. A study of the finer structure of the liver cell, made feasible by histochemistry, autoradiography, and electron microscopy, permits the detection of both early and late evidence of liver-cell damage. Repeat biopsies after treatment are helpful in a study of the influence of therapy on various parameters.

It is possible to determine by light microscopy whether a normal relationship between the liver cell and the sinusoids is present and to evaluate the appearance of individual liver cells. Special stains aid in the identification of fat, iron, glycogen, and other materials in the liver cell and allow the demonstration of damage reflected by altered cell size and staining, necrosis, and the presence of an inflammatory reaction. The location and character of the necrosis may be diagnostic. Thus, acidophilic coagulative necrosis is characteristic of virus hepatitis, hyaline necrosis is typically seen in alcoholic liver disease, and caseation necrosis is characteristic of tuberculosis (Figure 20).

It now appears that electron microscopy may aid in determining the cause of the changes seen by light microscopy. For example, mitochondrial enlargement and degeneration are characteristic of many malnourished alcoholics,[49] and repeat biopsies after treatment often show a reversion to normal. Changes in the activity of enzymes in the microsome following ingestion of common drugs are accompanied by alterations in

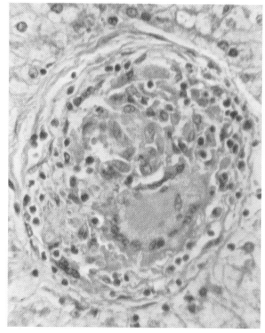

Figure 20. Tuberculous granulomatosis infiltration of liver. Liver biopsy may represent the best method for establishing a diagnosis of miliary tuberculosis. H&E (900x)

the structure of the smooth-surfaced endoplasmic reticulum. Decreases in drug-metabolizing enzyme activity (evoked by such drugs as iproniazid) may cause loss or vesiculation of the smooth endoplasmic reticulum, whereas increases in this activity (induced by such drugs as the barbiturates) are distinguished by proliferation of the smooth endoplasmic reticulum.[50] The presence of an unknown foreign pigment within the lysosome is characteristic of chronic idiopathic jaundice; on the other hand, copper and iron are found in these organelles in Wilson's disease and hemochromatosis respectively.

8

Functional Evaluation
of the Liver in Practice

Hepatic disease may initially involve a single physiologic-anatomic unit of the liver. However, most injurious agents ultimately involve all units. Therefore, it is usually necessary to evaluate simultaneously the functional state of the circulatory system, biliary network, reticuloendothelial cells, and liver cells. In this process, the clinician must, of necessity, be selective in his choice of laboratory studies. His objective should be to employ as few, simple, and inexpensive tests as possible for proper diagnosis and treatment.

Just which laboratory tests one should use depends upon whether one wishes to (1) identify subclinical hepatic abnormalities, (2) differentiate hepatic and extrahepatic causes of jaundice, (3) determine etiology, severity, and activity of overt liver disease, or (4) assess the regenerative potential of the diseased liver. Whenever possible, studies should be arranged to provide a complete diagnosis, including a designation of etiology, clinical status, biochemical-physiologic capacity, and morphologic changes (Box 11).

SUBCLINICAL LIVER DISEASE

Sensitive screening tests are necessary to detect subclinical liver diseases, that is, those not clinically evident. Their value is increased by the establishment of base-line (i.e., normal) hepatic patterns. The most certain way to identify hepatic alterations is to demonstrate cellular or subcellular *structural* changes in the liver. The most valuable biochemical test for identifying subclinical abnormalities is the bromsulfalein (BSP) test, particularly when blood samples are obtained at five, ten, and fifteen minutes (to allow calculation of the percentage disappearance rate) and at forty-five minutes (to provide insight into the dye's excretion). The cephalin flocculation and transaminase tests also are usually helpful in demonstrating the presence of active liver-cell damage.

JAUNDICE

It is usually easy to determine the mechanism responsible for uncomplicated jaundice. However, clinical problems do result because (1) it is difficult to differentiate between extrahepatic and intrahepatic causes of biliary obstruction, (2) continued extrahepatic obstruction leads to secondary liver-cell damage, and (3) two or more mechanisms may contribute simultaneously to hyperbilirubinemia.[51]

In a study of the jaundiced patient, it is first desirable to determine whether hyperbilirubinemia is due to (1) an increased production or deficient conjugation of bilirubin, (2) interference with secretion of bilirubin into biliary passages, or (3) interference with excretion of bilirubin. This may be accomplished by the use of four simple liver function tests—demonstration of bilirubin pigments in the urine, the cephalin flocculation test, and measurement of the serum alkaline phosphatase (Figure 21) and transaminases (Figure 22).

Unconjugated hyperbilirubinemia resulting from overproduction (hemolytic jaundice), faulty uptake, or lack of conjugation of bilirubin is not accompanied by significant

---

BOX 11

CLASSIFICATION OF LIVER DISEASE

The functional evaluation of the liver should be designed to provide a working diagnosis of hepatic disease. The following classification (similar to the one introduced by the American Heart Association for heart disease) provides a simple, practical approach to hepatic diagnosis.

A   Etiology

1. Nutritional deficiency and metabolic errors
   a. Imbalanced intake
   b. Abnormal absorption of food
   c. Abnormal assimilation of food
   d. Errors of metabolism

2. Toxic and infectious agents
   a. Chemicals and drugs
   b. Heavy metals
   c. Primary liver infections
   d. Secondary liver infections

3. Circulatory disturbances
   a. Passive congestion
   b. Hepatic vessel occlusion
   c. Diffuse vascular disease

4. Biliary obstruction
   a. Intrahepatic
   b. Extrahepatic

5. Neoplastic diseases

6. Trauma to liver

B   Clinical status

Grade   I. Subclinical liver abnormalities
Grade II. Compensated liver disease
Grade III. Liver disease with decompensation
Grade IV. Terminal liver disease

C   Biochemical-physiologic status

1. Excretory dysfunction
2. Metabolic functional impairment
3. Portal hypertension
4. Vascular shunts

D   Morphologic changes

1. Cellular alterations
   a. Fat deposit
   b. Fibrosis

anatomic alterations of any of the physiologic-anatomic units of the liver. Hemolytic jaundice is characterized by an increase in urine urobilinogen, no urine bilirubin, normal alkaline phosphatase and transaminases, and a negative cephalin flocculation test. Unconjugated hyperbilirubinemia due to faulty uptake (as is postulated for some forms of Gilbert's disease) or a defect in conjugation (as in the Crigler-Najjar syndrome) is accompanied by a normal urine urobilinogen.

Hyperbilirubinemia due to liver-cell damage (hepatocellular jaundice), however, is associated with alterations in each of the physiologic-anatomic units. Those tests which depend upon the integrity of the liver cell are primarily affected. Both bilirubin and urobilinogen may appear in the urine; the cephalin flocculation and transaminases are frequently abnormal. Although the serum alkaline phosphatase may be normal, it is often slightly elevated (see Figure 22, page 55).

---

   c. Regeneration
   d. Bile stasis
   e. Inflammation
   f. Liver-cell damage
   g. Necrosis
   h. Vascular changes
   i. Neoplasia
   j. Infiltrations
 2. Subcellular alterations in
   a. Nucleus
   b. Mitochondria
   c. Endoplasmic reticula—rough, smooth
   d. Lysosomes
   e. Biliary passages

The following classifications of a hypothetical jaundiced alcoholic with cirrhosis and a jaundiced patient having a common-duct stone illustrate the use of this schema.

Jaundiced alcoholic

A Etiology: Nutritional deficiency and alcoholism

B Clinical status: Grade III (decompensated)

C Biochemical-physiologic status:
   Excretory and metabolic dysfunction
   Portal hypertension and vascular shunts

D Morphologic changes:
   Fat 3+
   Fibrosis 3+
   Regeneration 3+
   Inflammation 2+
   Hyaline necrosis with mitochondrial swelling
      and degeneration
   Disruption of endoplasmic reticulum

Jaundiced patient with common-duct stone

A Etiology: Extrahepatic biliary obstruction due
   to calculi

B Clinical status: Grade II (compensated)

C Biochemical-physiologic status: Excretory
   dysfunction

D Morphologic changes: Bile stasis with portal
   inflammation and dilatation of bile canaliculi
   with atrophy of microvilli

In hyperbilirubinemia due to biliary obstruction (obstructive jaundice), bilirubin typically appears in the urine without urobilinogen, the serum alkaline phosphatase is increased, the cephalin flocculation remains normal, and the transaminases are normal or only slightly elevated.

After it has been decided that the basic cause of hyperbilirubinemia lies in one of these three categories, an attempt should be made to pinpoint the location and nature of the responsible lesion (Tables 3 and 4).

Unconjugated hyperbilirubinemia (increased production, decreased uptake, or deficient conjugation of bilirubin) — An increased production of bilirubin is most commonly seen in association with active destruction of circulating red cells, pulmonary infarction, hematomas, and transfusion of aged red cells. A sixfold increase in bilirubin production is not usually associated with a marked rise in serum bilirubin, since the normal liver excretes bilirubin in proportion to the square of the concentration in the serum. Hemolytic jaundice may be classified on the basis of its acuity or mechanism. Jaundice due to *acute* hemolysis is characterized by shock, hemoglobinuria, and various degrees of renal dysfunction, whereas decreased red-cell survival and reticulocytosis are prominent features in jaundice due to *chronic* hemolytic states.

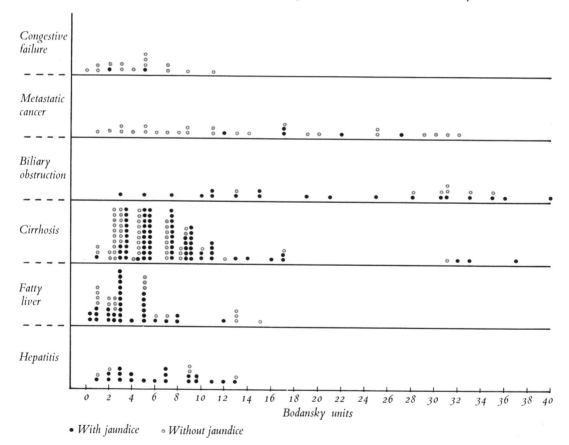

Figure 21. *Serum alkaline phosphatase in hepatic diseases.*

BILIRUBIN	URINARY PIGMENTS		CEPHALIN FLOCCULATION	ENZYMES	
	Urobilinogen	Bilirubin		Alk. Phosphatase	Transaminase
Increased production or deficient conjugation	+	o	o	o	o
Impaired secretion into biliary passage	±	±	+	o±	+
Impaired excretion	o	+	o	+	o±

o = absent or normal
+ = present or abnormal
± = borderline

Figure 22. Differential diagnosis of jaundice (hyperbilirubinemia).

Decreased uptake or lack of conjugation of bilirubin should be suspected in the infant or child with unconjugated hyperbilirubinemia. There are no detectable morphologic lesions on biopsy; the diagnosis is based on finding an increase in free (unconjugated) bilirubin, normal serum transaminase activity, absence of fecal stercobilinogen, and normal excretion of bromsulfalein.

A defect in transport of bilirubin from the serum to the area of the liver cell where it is conjugated has been suggested, although not proved, to be responsible for *constitutional hyperbilirubinemia*, or *Gilbert's disease*. This is a reasonably common asymptomatic state characterized by elevated free (unconjugated) serum bilirubin without an increase in conjugates, normal liver tissue on histologic examination, and normal biochemical liver function tests. The serum bilirubin rarely exceeds 5 to 7 mg. per 100 ml. The syndrome occurs in families and is inherited as a dominant characteristic. The hyperbilirubinemia of Gilbert's disease may increase with stress or infections and is occasionally accompanied by malaise and discomfort in the liver area. Patients with this condition are able to conjugate bilirubin as well as other substances, such as N-acetyl-*p*-aminophenol, menthol, and salicylamide, which are excreted as glucuronide conjugates.

A *lack of conjugation* of bilirubin is responsible for physiologic jaundice of the newborn, jaundice of immaturity, the Crigler-Najjar syndrome, jaundice in some newborn breast-fed infants, and icterus in premature infants receiving large doses of vitamin K analogues or certain antibiotics. In these conditions, a relative deficiency from inadequate synthesis or from competition for glucuronyl transferase and uridine diphosphate glucuronic acid dehydrogenase prevents conjugation. Physiologic jaundice of the newborn subsides rapidly, since the deficient enzymes appear soon after the first few days of life and there is a concomitant decrease in hemoglobin destruction. Withdrawal of breast feeding or vitamin K analogues (when these mechanisms are responsible for inhibiting conjugation of bilirubin)

Table 3

ANALYSIS OF A CASE OF HYPERBILIRUBINEMIA

Fractionate serum bilirubin and measure urine bilirubin and urobilinogen to determine whether:

I. Unconjugated hyperbilirubinemia.

Determine mechanism on basis of age, clinical features, and laboratory findings:

A. Production of bilirubin beyond excretory capacity. Evidence of:
  1. Hemolysis
     a. Extracorpuscular
        (1) Immune body reactions
           (a) Transfusion reactions
           (b) Erythroblastosis
        (2) Infections and chemicals
        (3) Physical agents
        (4) Secondary hemolysis in pregnancy
     b. Intracorpuscular
        (1) Congenital hemolytic jaundice
        (2) Sickle-cell anemia
        (3) Mediterranean anemia
  2. No hemolysis
     a. Pulmonary infarction
     b. Transfusion of aged red blood cells
     c. Hematomas
     d. "Shunt" hyperbilirubinemia

B. Deficient hepatic uptake of bilirubin:
  1. ? Gilbert's disease (normal biopsy, low-grade hyperbilirubinemia)
  2. ? Acquired liver disease

C. Deficient conjugation of bilirubin:
  1. Physiologic jaundice of newborn
     a. Inadequate bilirubin glucuronide synthesis
  2. Crigler-Najjar syndrome (transferase deficiency)
  3. Inhibition of glucuronyl transferase
     a. Large doses of vitamin K analogues in premature infants
     b. Increased level of pregnanediol
     c. Breast milk containing pregnane-3-(α), 20-(β)-diol
     d. Novobiocin

  a. Drugs detoxified as

II. Conjugated hyperbilirubinemia.
Determine mechanism on basis of age, clinical features, and laboratory findings:

A. Defect in bilirubin excretion. Confirm with serum alkaline phosphatase (elevated), cephalin flocculation (normal). In absence of rapid subsidence, exploratory surgery is desirable to differentiate:

  1. Extrahepatic biliary obstruction. Identify by radiologic means and/or direct inspection during surgical intervention
    a. Calculus
    b. Stricture
    c. Neoplasm

  2. Intrahepatic biliary obstruction. Confirm absence of extrahepatic biliary obstruction with operative or T-tube cholangiography. Identify localization of lesion by surgical biopsy
    a. Lesion of bile canaliculi   { (1) Drugs / (2) Viruses }
    b. Lesion of bile ductules   { (1) Drugs / (2) Viruses }
    c. Lesion of bile ducts   { (1) Drugs / (2) Viruses }

B. Deficient liver-cell secretion of bilirubin.
May need to differentiate from excretory defect by surgical exploration, cholangiography, or biopsy:

  1. Persistence of excretory defect in immature liver after development of adequate glucuronide-synthesizing capacity
  2. Dubin-Johnson syndrome (biopsy showing characteristic pigment)
  3. Rotor syndrome (absence of characteristic pigment)

III. Combined unconjugated and conjugated hyperbilirubinemia.
Determine mechanism on basis of clinical features and laboratory findings:

A. Familial defect or immature liver reflected in partial deficiency of glucuronide formation or excretion

B. Acquired liver-cell damage. Confirm with liver function tests and determine primary abnormality:
  1. Deficient hepatic uptake of bilirubin
  2. Deficient conjugation of bilirubin
  3. Deficient secretion or excretion of conjugated bilirubin

C. Hemolysis with secondary liver damage. Demonstrate presence of hemolysis:
  1. Hepatic damage secondary to shock
  2. Hepatic damage secondary to hemolysis

D. Biliary obstruction with secondary liver damage:
  1. Bile stasis with secondary injury
  2. Ascending cholangitis

likewise causes rapid subsidence of icterus. In contrast, unconjugated hyperbilirubinemia (usually quite marked) persists in the Crigler-Najjar syndrome, in which there is an inherited deficiency in transferase.

Conjugated hyperbilirubinemia (intrahepatic biliary cholestasis and extrahepatic biliary obstruction) — After bilirubin is conjugated in the liver cell, there may be interference with its secretion into the canaliculus or with its excretion once it reaches the canaliculus. Although the specific site of *excretory block* is not established in the congenital, intermittent, conjugated hyperbilirubinemia described by Dubin and Johnson, it would appear that the lesion may be precanalicular. In this condition, the liver cells contain a brown-black pigment which may cause general discoloration of the organ. Patients with the Dubin-Johnson syndrome frequently exhibit abdominal discomfort during episodes of increasing bilirubin. They may fail to excrete contrast media used for oral or intravenous cholangiography and have an abnormal excretion of bromsulfalein and indocyanine green. They exhibit a normal or only slightly elevated serum alkaline phosphatase. The closely related Rotor syndrome, which appears to represent a variant of the Dubin-Johnson syndrome, exhibits the same clinical features except that there is an absence of the liver pigment and a normal gall bladder is usually visualized.

Excretion of conjugated bilirubin may be interfered with by anatomic lesions demonstrable in the canaliculi, bile ductules, bile ducts, or extrahepatic biliary passages. In such cases, hyperbilirubinemia is commonly associated with an increase in the serum alkaline phosphatase and nonvisualization of the gall bladder on cholecystography. Atrophy of the microvilli of the canaliculi is characteristic in

intrahepatic cholestasis due to certain drugs, such as chlorpromazine and norethandrolone. In contrast, inflammatory lesions of the bile ductules and ducts represent the initial alteration in primary biliary cirrhosis. Biliary ob-

Table 4

Unconjugated Hyperbilirubinemia

Physiologic jaundice

Acquired postnatal

Rh incompatibility

"Shunt" hyperbilirubinemia

Gilbert's disease

Crigler-Najjar syndrome

Conjugated Hyperbilirubinemia

Extrahepatic biliary obstruction

Intrahepatic biliary obstruction

Dubin-Johnson syndrome

Rotor syndrome

Combined Hyperbilirubinemia

Neonatal hepatitis

Infectious hepatitis (viruses, bacteria, spirochetes, protozo
Metabolic disorders (glycogen, aminoaciduria, etc.)

struction beyond the liver may be caused by calculi, tumors, or bile-duct stricture.

It is essential to confirm the presence of conjugated hyperbilirubinemia by tests designed to demonstrate cholestasis or biliary obstruction. Cholestasis or biliary obstruction is frequently evident because of an elevated serum alkaline phosphatase and increased total serum cholesterol. Diagnosis is facilitated if functional study of the liver cell, by means of

DIFFERENTIAL DIAGNOSIS OF JAUNDICE IN INFANCY AND CHILDHOOD

Mechanism	Morphologic Findings	Biochemical Characteristics			Cholecystography or Cholangiography
		Serum Bilirubin	BSP Excretion		
Immaturity					
Drug or breast-milk inhibition of transferase activity					
Bilirubin overload	Bile stasis	Increased "indirect"	Normal		Normal
Bilirubin overload					
Familial defect in bilirubin uptake					
Familial deficiency in transferase activity					
Congenital defect	Bile stasis with or without intrahepatic ducts				Nonvisualization
Congenital defect	Bile stasis with or without intrahepatic ducts	Increased "direct"	Abnormal		Nonvisualization
Familial secretory defect	Pigmented liver cells				Variable
Familial excretory defect	Bile stasis without pigment				Visualization
Familial defect	Giant-cell hyperplasia				
Acquired	Evidence of liver-cell damage	Increased in both "direct" and "indirect"	Abnormal		Variable
Familial defect	Infiltration with glycogen, etc.				

such yardsticks as the cephalin flocculation test and serum cholesterol esters, shows no abnormality.

Differentiation of intrahepatic cholestasis and extrahepatic biliary obstruction may not be possible from clinical features and liver function tests. A diagnostic exploratory laparotomy is usually necessary when hyperbilirubinemia is persistent. Intrahepatic cholestasis is suggested by a history of the ingestion of drugs known to cause this condition (see Chapter 9, page 74). The diagnosis of extrahepatic biliary obstruction is favored by the existence of previous biliary surgery, fluctuation of serum bilirubin, distortion of the duodenum on barium study of the gastrointestinal tract, or failure to recover bile on duodenal drainage.

Mixed hyperbilirubinemia (hyperbilirubinemia due to a combination of decreased uptake, deficient conjugation, and/or decreased secretion of bilirubin) — Both conjugated and unconjugated serum bilirubin usually increase in instances of acquired liver-cell damage. There are also occasional chronically jaundiced patients who appear to have a familial defect in conjugation responsible for the accumulation of both types of bilirubin. The injured or necrotic liver cell may not be able to accept, store, conjugate, or secrete bilirubin into the biliary network. Moreover, increased production of unconjugated bilirubin may occur as a result of a shortened erythrocyte life span. The determination that liver-cell damage is responsible for the hyperbilirubinemia is based on the demonstration of cell dysfunction and the lack of evidence of biliary obstruction. This is often difficult, since liver-cell injury is frequently associated with obstruction to bile outflow, and biliary obstruction secondarily injures liver cells.

Studies of bilirubin metabolism in icterus due to *liver-cell damage* usually reveal increases in conjugated and unconjugated bilirubin, urine urobilinogen, and urine bilirubin. Urine urobilinogen studies are of special value since the appearance of this pigment decreases the likelihood of complete biliary obstruction. The serum alkaline phosphatase is of importance because a normal value reduces the probability that biliary obstruction is responsible for hyperbilirubinemia, although swelling of liver cells may interfere with excretion of this enzyme.

Determination of serum transaminase levels and results of the cephalin flocculation tests help to determine whether or not there is active liver-cell necrosis. Except in alcoholic fatty liver, a marked increase in serum transaminases occurs with liver-cell necrosis; the pyruvic tends to be more elevated than the oxalacetic transaminase in these instances.

The serum transaminases may be slightly increased because of an associated biliary obstruction. Typically, the oxalacetic is more elevated than the pyruvic transaminase in such cases. The cephalin flocculation test is frequently positive in instances of liver-cell damage but usually negative in early phases of biliary obstruction.

Liver biopsy is the most important diagnostic procedure in patients with hyperbilirubinemia due to hepatic damage. It confirms the presence of liver-cell damage and provides the only certain method for differentiating hepatitis, fatty liver, cirrhosis, and infiltrative lesions.

HEPATITIS

Acute inflammation and necrosis of the liver may result from a variety of infective agents, drugs, or chemicals. Laboratory studies are desirable not only to establish the cause of the inflammation but also to assess the severity of the hepatitis and to determine when healing has occurred.

The "virus of hepatitis" is the most common cause of liver inflammation (Box 12). The illness it produces is usually readily recognized when it occurs in epidemic forms; however, considerable diagnostic difficulty is presented by isolated cases. The physician's problems would be greatly facilitated by a simple, readily available method of demonstrating the infective agent. Unfortunately, the current inability to culture the virus and the lack of a reliable serologic test mean that recognition of "virus hepatitis" depends upon circumstantial evidence. A history of exposure to another patient with hepatitis or parenteral injections of blood or its products are important clues. An attempt should be made to elicit a history of contact with drugs or exposure to chemicals that may cause liver damage (Table 5).

An enlarged and tender liver suggests the presence of acute hepatitis. Biochemical liver function tests permit the confirmation of hepatitis and the assessment of its severity and degree of activity. The most valuable diagnostic tests are the serum transaminases. Both the serum glutamic oxalacetic and pyruvic transaminases are usually increased above 400 units (normal is 40 units) during the initial phases of hepatitis, the pyruvic being slightly higher than the oxalacetic transaminase. The activities of these enzymes increase in the serum because of their release from the damaged liver cell. There is a gradual decrease with recovery. (A decrease may also occur in the absence of healing in patients with autolytic necrosis or those treated with adrenal steroids.)

The serum alkaline phosphatase is also valuable in diagnosis since it may permit the differentiation of hepatitis from intrahepatic cholestasis and extrahepatic biliary obstruc-

Table 5

SOME DRUGS AND CHEMICALS
CAUSING LIVER-CELL DAMAGE
BY DIRECT TOXIC REACTION

Amanita phalloides toxin
Arsenic
Beryllium
Carbon tetrachloride
Chloroform
Ferrous sulfate
Phosphorus
Trinitrotoluene

tion. This enzyme may be normal or increased in hepatitis. An elevated alkaline phosphatase may result from swelling of the liver cell, with secondary pressure on finer biliary passages. It may also be due to primary injury of the biliary canaliculi or ductules.

The serum bilirubin concentration provides an objective means of measuring the degree of hyperbilirubinemia; ancillary studies, such as the urine urobilinogen and urine bilirubin, may provide the first clues to the presence of hepatic disease. Although biochemical tests alone may be sufficient in the average patient with hepatitis, they should be supplemented by liver biopsy in cases of atypical, persistent, or severe hepatitis.

Serial studies are desirable in patients with hepatitis to determine when the inflammatory process has subsided. They are particularly helpful in patients with persistent or chronic hepatitis. During the icteric phase of hepatitis, serum transaminases and serum bilirubin provide the minimal information needed. After subsidence of icterus, serum transaminases and bromsulfalein removal should be studied until abnormalities disappear. Patients with persistent hepatitis should have a liver biopsy and special blood studies, including electrophoretic protein patterns.

A large number of other infective agents may primarily or secondarily involve the liver. In these instances, it is important to establish the etiologic diagnosis, since the effects on the liver are quite similar (Table 6).

FATTY LIVER AND OTHER METABOLIC ALTERATIONS

Enlargement of the liver and alteration in its function may result from fatty metamorphosis, excess glycogen deposition, and accumulation of iron, copper, amyloid, or abnormal lipid. The history, physical examination, and laboratory tests may suggest the presence of these conditions; however, liver biopsy provides the only certain means of relating hepatic abnormalities to the metabolic alterations. The accumulation of such materials within the cell may cause displacement of its nucleus and may alter the functions of various subcellular organelles within the cytoplasm.

Fatty liver probably is the most frequent of all hepatic alterations. This condition results from increased deposition of fat in the liver (transport or synthesis), altered removal of hepatic lipids (transport or oxidation), or a combination of these factors. It is most commonly seen in patients who are ingesting

---

BOX 12

VIRUS HEPATITIS

A variety of viruses may cause hepatitis; the most common were originally designated IH, or A, and SH, or B. IH (for "infectious hepatitis"), or A, virus is transmitted by oral-intestinal contamination but may be spread by parenteral means, whereas SH (for "serum hepatitis"), or B, virus is transmitted only by parenteral means. Recently, virologists have cultured viruses (AR 17) which, when given to human volunteers, have apparently reproduced this disease. Three basic pathologic lesions are encountered in virus hepatitis: (1) localized necrosis, (2) functional alterations of the bile canaliculi with or without pericholangiolitis, and (3) massive, or autolytic, necrosis.

In virus hepatitis with localized necrosis, the liver-cell nucleus becomes pyknotic and the cytoplasm eosinophilic. A hyaline mass is formed and is extruded into the space of Disse. This process is accompanied by intralobular and periportal inflammation. Cytolysosomes and altered endoplasmic reticula are characteristic on electron microscopy. With severe injury, the mitochondria swell and disintegrate. There is active proliferation of mesenchymal, ductular, and liver cells on serial study. The localized necrosis of virus hepatitis contrasts sharply with lesions seen in primary cholangiolar involvement or autolytic necrosis. In the latter state, there is complete disappearance of recognizable liver cells in entire lobules.

Normally, virus hepatitis heals within three months, and there is no residuum. Persistent virus hepatitis with continuing clinical and laboratory evidence of an active disease may be due to a delay in healing, perhaps because of the development of an autoimmune reaction or a persisting infection. Unavailability of practical clinical methods for identifying the virus of hepatitis makes it impossible to determine which of these mechanisms is responsible in most patients with persistent hepatitis. An

inadequate amounts of protein because of its unavailability or as a result of alcoholism, chronic illness, or food fads (Figure 23).

Fatty liver is manifested by a variable symptom complex which may simulate an acute surgical abdomen or obstructive jaundice and produce manifestations of portal hypertension or symptoms of acute hepatic failure. Morphologic studies reveal various amounts of liver fat, often associated with enlarged and degenerated mitochondria. A fatty liver is frequently accompanied by abnormal liver function tests (Figure 24), multiple vitamin deficiencies, blood sugar disturbances, ane-mia, and renal abnormalities attributable to a combination of hepatic injury and nutritional deficiency. Early recognition and treatment of this completely reversible condition is desirable; the progress of fat mobilization may best be followed by serial biopsies.

Increased amounts of liver *glycogen* are commonly seen in diabetes; indeed, massive amounts often accumulate and produce transient hepatomegaly in patients being treated for diabetic coma. The resulting hepatomegaly may cause abnormal tenderness or anorexia. There may be BSP retention and other abnormalities of liver function.

---

autoimmune reaction has received most attention and has been assumed to be present because of the marked increase in gamma globulin, evidence of other features of an immunologic abnormality, and dramatic improvement following adrenal steroid therapy.

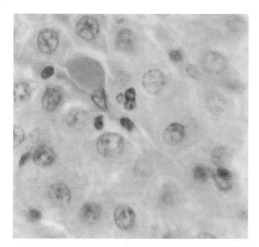

Microscopic section from a thirty-year-old laborer with acute virus hepatitis, showing eosinophilic coagulative necrosis. H&E (1200x)

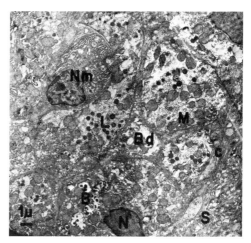

Electron micrograph from a patient with acute virus hepatitis, showing fractionation of the endoplasmic reticulum into small vesicles; collapse of reticulum fibers, "C"; bile within the parenchyma, "B"; a mesenchymal cell, "Nm"; bile ductules, "Bd"; and cellular debris in the sinusoid, "S."

Table 6

CHARACTERISTICS OF INFECTIVE AGENTS
COMMONLY RESPONSIBLE FOR LIVER DAMAGE

Disease	*Hepatic Lesion*	*Other Lesions*	*Specific Laboratory Diagnosis*
Virus hepatitis A	Liver-cell necrosis		
Virus hepatitis B	Liver-cell necrosis		
Infectious mononucleosis	Liver-cell necrosis	Pharyngitis, lymphadenitis	Heterophil agglutination
Yellow fever	Liver-cell necrosis	Hemoglobinemia, nephrosis	Isolate organism from urine, complement-fixation test, mouse protection test, histologic examination of postmortem specimen
Tuberculosis	Miliary lesions, tuberculoma, tuberculous lymphadenopathy	Pulmonary, gastro-intestinal tuberculosis, etc.	Culture of liver biopsy, demonstration of acid-fast bacilli
Brucellosis	Granuloma	Systemic infection	Blood culture, culture of liver biopsy, agglutination studies
Typhoid fever	Focal necrosis	Gastro-intestinal lesions	Blood culture
Syphilis	Gummas, interstitial hepatitis	Generalized infection	Treponema pallidum immobilization test, complement-fixation test
Leptospirosis	Liver-cell necrosis	Renal necrosis	Blood culture, animal inoculation, agglutination titer
Amebiasis	Hepatitis or liver abscess	Intestinal lesions	Stool and aspirate examination
Echinococcosis	Formation of hepatic cysts	Intestinal lesions	Scolices in stool, skin test
Schistosomiasis	Hepatic granuloma, pipestem fibrosis	Intestinal lesions	Rectal biopsy, liver biopsy
Clonorchiasis	Cholangitis, cirrhosis	Intestinal lesions	Ova in stools or duodenal drainage

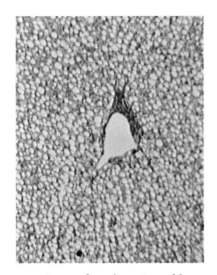

Figure 23. Severe fatty liver in a fifty-year-old woman with uncontrolled diabetes. H&E (250x)

A variety of genetically induced defects in carbohydrate metabolism lead to excess liver glycogen. The most frequent is a deficiency of glucose 6-phosphatase, an enzyme necessary for glycogenolysis.[52] This condition is usually characterized by an enlarged liver, symptoms incident to hypoglycemia, and a low blood sugar that is not altered by epinephrine or glucagon. Liver biopsy will confirm the presence of increased glycogen and may help identify the enzymatic deficiency. Closely related is the inborn absence of an enzyme, uridine diphosphogalactose (elegantly abbreviated as UDP-Gal) transferase, which is necessary for conversion of galactose to glucose. The resulting galactosemia is accompanied by weight loss, hepatomegaly, various degrees of hepatic failure, aminoaciduria, cataracts, and mental deficiency. The lesions consist in fatty or fibrotic changes in addition to excess glycogen in parenchymal cells. A spectrophotometric test in which erythrocytes from galactosemic subjects are incubated with galactose demonstrates an accumulation of galactose phosphate.[53]

Marked hepatic abnormalities occur in *amyloidosis*. This condition has been classified into a primary and secondary variety on the basis of etiology, position of the organ, and affinity of the deposits for special stains. However, either group may have hepatic infiltration with amyloid. In the liver, this glycoprotein is deposited between the endothelial cells of the sinusoids and may cause compression atrophy of liver cells. In the primary variety, deposition is mainly around the arteries. The clinical features may be due to involvement of the liver or other organs. Biochemical liver function tests are usually only slightly deranged.

Three eponymic disorders—Letterer-Siwe's disease, Gaucher's disease, and Niemann-Pick's disease—are frequently associ-

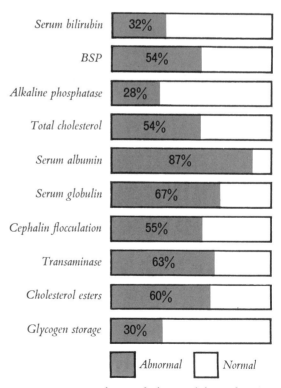

Figure 24. Incidence of abnormal liver function tests in fatty liver.

ated with hepatic alterations caused by the accumulation of *abnormal lipids* in the liver. The diagnosis of these disorders depends upon identification of the abnormal lipid, the presence of a normal serum cholesterol, and the clinical features characteristic of the disease (Table 7).

The accumulation of excess hepatic iron and copper is characteristic of *hemosiderosis* and Wilson's disease respectively. Much attention has been directed recently to excess iron accumulation, since it has been shown that a large number of patients with liver disease have an increased hepatic content of this metal (Figure 25). Iron may accumulate because of (1) excess ingestion, with resultant increased intestinal absorption, (2) an inborn error that allows absorption in greater amounts than needed, or (3) an acquired gastro-intestinal alteration that facilitates excess absorption. Circulating iron may also be deposited in the liver when it is given parenterally, following multiple transfusions, or as a result of chronic hemolysis. Iron is observed in both Kupffer and parenchymal cells, where it accumulates in the mitochondria and lysosomes (Figure 26, Table 8). Although excess iron may appear in other organs, the liver is the chief repository. Serial liver biopsy is the best method for evaluating the effectiveness of treatment of this condition, which may be greatly improved by depletion of body iron.[54]

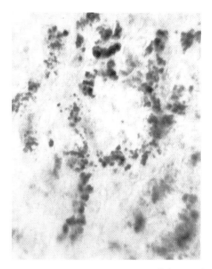

Figure 25. Microscopic section of liver from a patient with diabetes, skin pigmentation, and evidence of liver failure showing marked deposition of iron. Prussian blue stain (900x)

Liver lesions are often the most prominent features of *Wilson's disease*, or hepatolenticular degeneration. This condition is characterized by the triad of basal ganglia degeneration, pigmentation of Descemet's membrane of the limbus of the cornea, and hepatic fibrosis. The lesions have been attributed to persistent aminoaciduria, disturbances in copper metabolism, and an unknown toxin. Abnormal copper metabolism appears to be the major defect leading to other alterations. Patients with Wilson's disease show increased absorp-

Table 7

LIPID HISTOCYTOSIS INVOLVING LIVER

Disease	Biochemical Alteration
Letterer-Siwe's disease	Accumulation of cholesterol secondary to granulomatous lesions
Gaucher's disease	Accumulation of kerasin due to inborn error
Niemann-Pick's disease	Accumulation of sphingomyelin due to inborn error

Table 8

IRON-STORAGE DISEASE

	Idiopathic "Familial" Hemochromatosis	Transfusion Hemosiderosis	Hemosiderosis Secondary to Absorption Abnormality or Excess Dietary Iron
Serum iron	Increased	Normal	Normal or Increased
Unsaturated iron binding	1-2+	1-2+	0-1+
Insulin insufficiency	2-4+	1+	1+
Hepatic iron distribution	Parenchymal cells	Kupffer cells	Parenchymal and Kupffer cells
Hemofuscin	2+	2+	2+
Iron absorption	1-4+	1-4+	1-4+
Hepatic fibrosis	1-4+	2+	2+

tion of copper from the gastro-intestinal tract, decreased serum alpha-2-globulin-bound copper (this form of copper protein is blue in the purified state and has been named "ceruloplasmin"), increased serum albumin-bound copper, and excess tissue copper.

Wilson's disease should be suspected when signs of basal ganglion dysfunction are present in a patient with evidence of hepatic disease. Aminoaciduria, increased urinary excretion of copper, and decreased serum ceruloplasmin are diagnostic. The clinical and laboratory abnormalities related to the liver depend upon morphologic alterations; these may range from fatty liver to diffuse fibrosis or postnecrotic cirrhosis. Increased pericanalicular dense bodies and reduced liver-cell acid phosphatase activity are often noted on the electron microscope.[55] Many patients with terminal Wilson's disease exhibit evidence of liver failure, including icterus, ascites, hepatic fetor, and bleeding esophageal varices.

CIRRHOSIS

Cirrhosis should always be suspected in pa-

tients with signs of liver failure. It is a more tenable postulate when palpation reveals hardening of this organ, but absolute proof de-

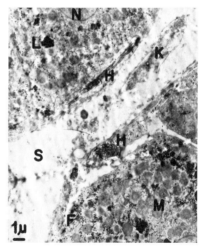

Figure 26. Electron micrograph of a section of liver from a patient with hemochromatosis. "H" shows hemosiderin in the space of Disse with part of a Kupffer cell, "K," in the sinusoid, "S." Note the intracellular ferritin that appears as small black dots throughout the cells and its concentration in the lysosomes, "L." (8000x)

BOX 13

CIRRHOSIS

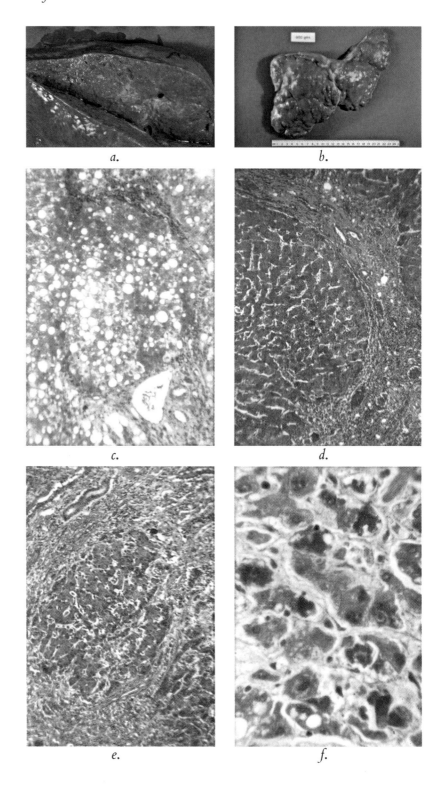

a.

b.

c.

d.

e.

f.

The term "cirrhosis" has a number of connotations. However, it is best used to indicate distortion of hepatic lobular architecture. Since lobular distortion is accompanied by various degrees of liver-cell dysfunction and intrasinusoidal hypertension, this definition includes both morphologic and clinical features. Lesions which initially involve a single physiologic-anatomic unit of the liver often ultimately lead to cirrhosis with involvement of all units.

Laennec's and postnecrotic cirrhosis begin with destruction of the liver cell. These types of cirrhosis overlap and may be produced by a variety of different etiologic factors. Classically, Laennec's cirrhosis is characterized by a finely nodular liver which is the seat of diffuse fibrosis, pseudolobules, and bile-duct proliferation, with or without fatty metamorphosis. In contrast, surface nodulation is irregular in postnecrotic cirrhosis, and there are wider bands of connective tissue which contain two or more portal tracts. Features of both types of cirrhosis often occur in the same person. Fine structural studies demonstrate proliferation of bile ductules, a mesenchymal reaction, and fibrogenesis in both Laennec's and postnecrotic cirrhosis. Laennec's cirrhosis is usually a sequel to chronic alcoholism. Ethanol causes liver-cell damage in the setting of malnutrition, and the resulting necrosis evokes a proliferative reaction of mesenchymal, ductular, and liver cells.

Postnecrotic cirrhosis results either from continued single-cell and "piecemeal" necrosis or from massive autolytic necrosis. Piecemeal necrosis may be due to a variety of mechanisms; it slowly causes liver-cell destruction with a regenerative response that accounts for the morphologic findings. Massive autolysis, usually associated with severe virus or toxic hepatitis, often involves an entire lobule, causes collapse fibrosis, and simultaneously produces a regenerative response.

Lesions of the biliary tract initially cause bile-duct proliferation and fibrosis primarily involving the biliary tract. Continuation of this process ultimately evokes a general regenerative response with production of cirrhosis. Similarly, chronic circulatory congestion associated with heart failure, veno-occlusive disease, or hepatic vein thrombosis at first produces pericentral vein fibrosis which later may be transformed into a generalized process.

Cardiac fibrosis is very frequent in patients with chronic circulatory congestion. Cirrhosis in patients with heart failure usually seems to be attributable to mechanisms other than circulatory congestion, but it may occur following constrictive pericarditis, tricuspid incompetence, or veno-occlusive disease.

a. Gross section of liver from alcoholic with Laennec's cirrhosis. Characteristic fine, uniform nodulation. b. Liver of man with posthepatitis (postnecrotic) cirrhosis. Large nodules vary in size. c. Periportal fibrosis with fat in early cirrhosis of the alcoholic. May show few clinical and laboratory abnormalities. d. Hyperplastic lobule surrounded by connective tissue with inflammatory cells. Lesions due to postnecrotic changes. Seen in over half of alcoholics with established cirrhosis. e. Diffuse fibrosis with pseudolobules devoid of central vein, typical of Laennec's cirrhosis. f. Hyaline necrosis (red) and fat frequently accompanied by jaundice, leukocytosis, and fever.

(From Leevy, C. M.: Practical Diagnosis and Treatment of Liver Disease. New York: Paul B. Hoeber, Inc., 1957. Courtesy of the author and publisher)

pends upon morphologic studies. Whenever possible, liver biopsy should be performed to confirm the diagnosis of cirrhosis and to establish its type, severity, activity, and regenerative capacity (Box 13).

After the diagnosis of cirrhosis is established, it is desirable to assess the biochemical status by means of liver function tests and to perform physiologic studies to determine whether portal hypertension is present. Results of such studies provide helpful data to support a diagnosis of cirrhosis in patients in whom biopsy is not possible. The choice of liver function tests should depend upon the absence or presence of the complications of cirrhosis; in their absence, the clinical work-up should include determinations of serum bilirubin (if the patient is jaundiced), bromsulfalein excretion (in the absence of jaundice), serum protein electrophoresis, cephalin flocculation, and serum transaminases. Since portal hypertension is usually present, it is desirable to perform esophagoscopy or barium study of the esophagus to verify the existence of esophageal varices. The actual portal pressure may be measured indirectly by the technics of splenic pulp puncture or wedged hepatic vein catheterization.[11]

Special laboratory tests are necessary for patients who have the complications of cirrhosis, i.e., gastro-intestinal bleeding, mental changes, ascites, or renal dysfunction. Gastrointestinal bleeding constitutes the most important and devastating of these complications. In the majority of instances, it is due to rupture of esophageal varices; but it is necessary to localize the site of hemorrhage since it may also occur from other mechanisms (peptic ulcers are the second most frequent cause of intestinal hemorrhage in these patients). This is possible by endoscopy, use of a modified string test employing the recently available Diagnostotube,[6] and barium stud-

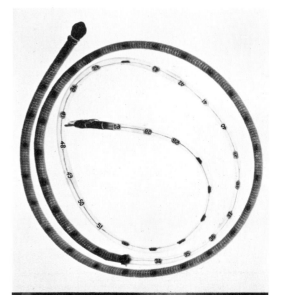

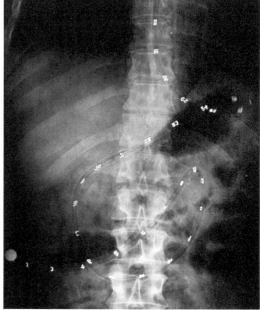

Figure 27. The Diagnostotube—detailed view and appearance on x-ray.

ies of the upper gastro-intestinal tract. The Diagnostotube is particularly valuable in localizing the site of bleeding in patients with active hemorrhage (Figure 27). The advantages of the Diagnostotube technic over the conventional string test include the following: (1) It is easily introduced, (2) an anatomical site is exactly located by a number rather than by a linear marker, (3) curling of the tube within the stomach does not interfere with localization, (4) the tube may be reused after each examination if the sheath is changed. Measurement of the blood ammonia, BSP removal, and splenic pressure are not helpful in differential diagnosis in patients with established liver disease; the results are usually abnormal in cirrhosis with intestinal bleeding, regardless of the source of hemorrhage.

Each patient with cirrhosis should be evaluated for mental changes. Neuropsychiatric examination frequently reveals evidence of hepatic encephalopathy that may result from a variety of conditions, including abnormal protein metabolism, hypoglycemia, electrolyte disturbances, and primary vascular changes.

An elevated blood ammonia is characteristic of hepatic encephalopathy; this has led to the belief that ammonium intoxication or another, as yet unidentified, abnormality in protein metabolism is responsible for that state. Nevertheless, some patients (perhaps 10 percent) with elevated ammonia levels do not exhibit overt mental changes, whereas others (10 percent) with a normal ammonia level have profound neuropsychiatric abnormalities. As shown on page 18, interference with the synthesis of urea from ammonia (which leads to increased ammonia levels) may result either from deficient hepatic function or from portal collateral circulation which allows intestinal products to bypass the liver. The large intestine is the principal site of ammonia production; however, variable amounts enter the circulation from the stomach, the upper intestinal tract, and the kidneys. In addition, potassium deficiency may contribute to an elevation of blood ammonia and its symptom complex. There is also, characteristically, a slowing of the electroencephalogram in patients with hepatic encephalopathy, the degree of abnormality often paralleling a rise in arterial ammonia.[56]

Serial blood ammonia levels and electroencephalographic studies are useful objective means of evaluating the effectiveness of therapy. Restricted ingestion of ammonia-producing foods and use of antibiotics to decrease intestinal production of urea-splitting bacteria are necessary to control ammonium intoxication in patients with severe liver disease. Their response to the ingestion of the standard (60-Gm.) protein test meal (described on page 48) helps the physician decide on the need for continuing one or both of these forms of therapy.

The procedures described above are designed to facilitate use of supportive measures available for managing the patient with complications of cirrhosis. In-vitro studies of DNA synthesis (page 39) in percutaneous biopsy specimens from patients with a progressively deteriorating cirrhosis indicate that liver failure may result from a deficiency of the enzymes and substrates necessary for hepatic regeneration. In-vivo correction of a folic acid, pyridoxine, or vitamin B_{12} deficiency restores in-vitro DNA synthesis to normal and initiates clinical and laboratory improvement.[57] Therefore, it is desirable for the clinician to assess the regenerative capacity in subjects with cirrhosis who fail to respond to supportive therapy and to identify and correct deficiencies of nucleogenic vitamins, trace metals, and other substances which are of critical importance to nucleic acid synthesis.

Electrolyte and renal studies are required in addition to hepatic tests for the proper treatment of ascites, electrolyte imbalance, or kidney failure, which frequently complicate liver disease. A diagnostic paracentesis and other laboratory tests are desirable to differentiate ascites due to hepatic disorders from that caused by metastatic cancer, tuberculous peritonitis, or constrictive pericarditis. In patients with azotemia, studies of urinary sediment, renal function tests, and, in selected instances, kidney biopsy are necessary to differentiate primary renal disease from terminal liver disease, in which there is often a decrease in glomerular filtration rate and renal blood flow. Observations in the Jersey City Medical Center indicate that approximately 20 percent of patients with cirrhosis and renal impairment have pyelonephritis or glomerulonephritis; 60 percent have prerenal azotemia resulting from hypotension and shock incident to such conditions as gastro-intestinal hemorrhage or electrolyte imbalance; and approximately 20 percent have renal dysfunction of unknown origin that is characterized by a decrease in renal blood flow and an increase in renal vascular resistance.

The availability of thiazides, spirolactones, and other potent diuretic agents has improved the control of ascites but has also increased the incidence of electrolyte imbalance and renal failure. Responsiveness to sodium restriction and diuretics should be monitored by daily measurement of body weight, abdominal girth, and urinary excretion of sodium to determine the effectiveness of a diuretic regimen and to minimize complications. A combination of studies of pH, plasma volume, serum sodium, serum potassium, and serum chloride provides adequate orientation to select appropriate corrective therapy for acid-base and electrolyte disturbances.

NEOPLASTIC LESIONS

The liver is frequently the site of both benign and malignant tumors. Hemangiomas and nonparasitic cysts occasionally produce hepatomegaly, pain, and other symptoms. Percutaneous needle biopsy should not be employed in such lesions because of the possibility of hemorrhage.

Recognition of metastatic cancer in the

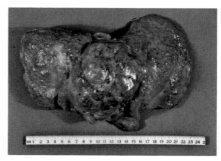

Gross appearance

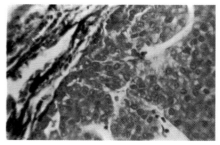

Microscopic section
Trichrome stain (250x)

Figure 28. Hepatoma in a patient with chronic alcoholism who was followed for eight years. Serial biopsies showed Laennec's cirrhosis with development of postnecrotic features. Progressive enlargement of the liver and onset of ascites accompanied by an increase in serum alkaline phosphatase appeared during the last two years of life.

liver in its early phases constitutes a difficult and frequently impossible task. In its later phases, it may be suspected from the presence of a nodular liver, by an increase in serum alkaline phosphatase, or by a rarefied area on photoscans. Morphologic proof can be obtained through biopsy at the site of rarefaction. Lesions less than 2 cm. in diameter do not reveal themselves on photoscans and are rarely penetrated by blind biopsy.

Primary cancer of the liver is often superimposed on cirrhosis (Figure 28). The incidence of hepatoma in cirrhosis of the alcoholic ranges from 4 to 9 percent, in postnecrotic cirrhosis from 8 to 15 percent, and in hemochromatosis from 15 to 20 percent. Progression of hepatomegaly and weight loss, increase of serum alkaline phosphatase, and pain from bone metastases are suggestive clinical features

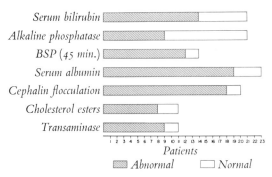

Figure 29. Biochemical liver function tests in twenty-three alcoholic patients with cirrhosis and primary liver cancer encountered over a twelve-year period in the Jersey City Medical Center.

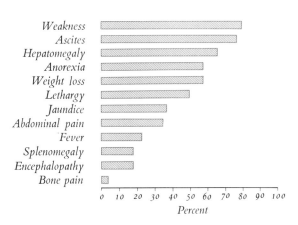

Figure 30. Clinical features in twenty-six alcoholic patients with cirrhosis and primary liver cancer encountered over a twelve-year period in the Jersey City Medical Center.

(Figures 29 and 30). Photoscanning combined with needle biopsy may facilitate detection of malignancy superimposed on cirrhosis. The autoradiographic technic (described on page 39) employing in-vitro tritiated thymidine shows marked labeling of neoplastic liver cells; this finding may facilitate differentiation of cancerous and noncancerous regenerative hyperplasia.

9

Drug-Induced Liver Injury

The historical assignment of a key role to the liver in drug metabolism is justified by current observations which indicate that (1) the liver is a major site for storage, detoxification, and excretion of drugs; (2) liver dysfunction may interfere with metabolism of a drug and thereby lead to untoward pharmacologic effects; (3) some drugs in clinical use occasionally cause damage to the liver; (4) use of a large number of valuable therapeutic agents must be restricted or prohibited because of hepatotoxicity.

Each year there become available an increasing number of new pharmacologic preparations whose hepatic metabolism and hepatotoxicity must be investigated and defined. The practicing physician must therefore be aware of the potential untoward effects of these agents on the liver and be prepared to detect undesirable hepatic reactions even in the absence of previous documentation of such problems.

ROLE OF THE LIVER IN DRUG METABOLISM

By means of radioisotopic preparations, drug uptake and storage by the human liver and excretory maximal tubular capacity (Tm) have been established for a limited number of pharmacologic agents. Such measurements provide another important and practical parameter for determining the effect of liver injury on drug metabolism. Hepatic uptake has been determined from plasma disappearance rates; storage has been estimated through comparison of the hepatic tissue and circulating levels of drugs; and biliary excretion has been evaluated by serial study of drug concentration in the serum and bile.[58] Storage and excretory transport maximums may also be determined indirectly by comparing the rate of movement of a substance into the liver with different rates of change in its concentration in the plasma.[59]

Many drugs, as typified by cortisol,[60] are selectively removed from the circulation by the liver following parenteral administration; their half-life depends upon the rate of uptake by the liver. Hepatic uptake, storage, and release are also the chief factors which regulate circulating levels of drugs that enter the portal circulation after oral ingestion. The disposition of those drugs which are concentrated in the liver varies considerably. Some are stored for long periods of time in the Kupffer cells;[58] many are excreted as water-soluble conjugates and often undergo an enterohepatic circulation.[61]

EFFECT OF HEPATIC DYSFUNCTION ON DRUG METABOLISM

Inability of the severely impaired liver to store, metabolize, or excrete a drug may greatly exaggerate its pharmacologic effects. This has been best documented in the case of barbiturates and morphine.[62] For example, an average therapeutic amount of either of these agents may cause marked sensorial or respiratory depression or coma in the patient with liver failure. On the other hand, such drugs are usually well tolerated by patients with compensated liver disease. Blood levels, biliary excretion, and urinary excretion of drugs that are normally stored or metabolized in the liver are often significantly altered when there is a reduced hepatic blood flow, a decrease in the number of healthy liver cells, or an obstruction to bile outflow. Intrahepatic vascular shunts may cause notable changes in drug metabolism, as illustrated by studies of oral sulfonylurea derivatives. These agents have a much more pronounced effect on peripheral glucose in patients with cirrhosis and vascular shunts than in subjects with a normal liver.[63] Also, substances like glucagon, which exercises a primary pharmacologic effect within the liver, usually produce quantitatively different reactions in the presence of liver disease. Therefore, the degree of glucagon-induced hyperglycemia is less and hepatic oxygen consumption is relatively greater when there is cirrhosis than when the liver is normal.[64] In the absence of liver failure, a deficiency of transferase or an alteration in microsomal mechanisms for detoxification may interfere with disposition of such drugs as chloramphenicol, morphine, certain barbiturates, benzedrine, codeine, aniline, progesterone, thyroxine, and tetrahydrocortisone.

MECHANISM OF DRUG-INDUCED HEPATOTOXICITY

Hepatic damage produced by drugs may result from a direct toxic effect or from a hypersensitivity reaction[65,66] (Tables 9, 10, and 11). Drugs which produce *direct* hepatic toxicity are considered to be protoplasmic poisons. Their effects may result from injury of selected organelles within the liver cell or bile passages or from inhibition of metabolites essential for specific organelle function. The localization of the lesion depends upon the drug; for example, carbon tetrachloride causes mitochondrial and microsomal injury, whereas anabolic steroids may produce atrophy of the microvilli of the canaliculi. Direct hepatotoxicity is predictable and is characterized by (1) a brief interval between exposure and the development of liver damage, (2) a toxicity

Table 9

SOME DRUGS CAUSING INTRAHEPATIC BILIARY OBSTRUCTION (CHOLESTASIS) BY DIRECT TOXIC REACTION

17α-ethyl-17-hydroxynorandrostenone (norethandrolone) (Nilevar®)

17α-ethinyl-19-nortestosterone (norethindrone) (Norlutin®)

1-dehydro-17α-methyltestosterone (methandrostenolone) (Dianabol®)

9α-fluoro-11β-hydroxy-17-methyltestosterone (fluoxymesterone) (Halotestin®)

19-nor-17β-hydroxy-3-keto-androstene-17-phenylpropionate (nandrolone phenpropionate) (Durabolin®)

which is related to the dose, and (3) a similar and reproducible condition in experimental animals.

Table 10

SOME DRUGS CAUSING LIVER-CELL DAMAGE BY HYPERSENSITIVITY REACTION OR METABOLIC IDIOSYNCRASY

Incidence

> 1 percent	Carbutamide (BZ-55) Halothane (Fluothane®) Iproniazid (Marsilid®) 6-Mercaptopurine (Purinethol®) Phenacemide (Phenurone®) Triacetyloleandomycin (TAO®) Zoxazolamine (Flexin®) DDT Synthalin®
< 1 percent	Chlorambucil (Leukeran®) Chloramphenicol (Chloromycetin®) Diphenylhydantoin (Dilantin®) Mephenytoin (Mesantoin®) Phenindione (Hedulin®) Phenylbutazone (Butazolidin®) Trimethadione (Tridione®) Cinchophen Aminosalicylic acid (PAS) Tetracyclines Urethan

Drug-induced *hypersensitivity* reactions within the liver may result from allergy when the pharmacologic agent acts as a haptene and evokes production of an antibody that remains attached to the cells; on the other hand, the reaction may represent individual metabolic susceptibility to specific drug toxicity. The composition of a compound determines, in part, its capacity to sensitize; for example, chlorine-containing drugs are notable for their ability to cause hypersensitivity reactions.

Drug reactions involving the liver have certain characteristics. The incidence is low in man; their occurrence in any given individual is unpredictable and is not related to dosage; cross-sensitization, desensitization, or hyposensitization may be produced. Unfortunately, such reactions are *not* detectable by any known means in animal studies. In contrast to the fixed area of injury that is usually characteristic of drugs causing direct toxic effects, the location of the site of injury in the liver varies considerably with drugs which produce hypersensitivity reactions. Chlorpromazine (which appears to cause hepatotoxicity by this mechanism) may primarily involve the liver cell, the biliary passages, or both in a given individual.

MANIFESTATIONS OF DRUG-INDUCED HEPATOTOXICITY

Drugs or chemicals that cause direct toxic effects or produce hypersensitivity reactions may adversely affect one or more of the four physiologic-anatomic units of the liver. Most often they produce liver-cell damage, lesions of the biliary passages, or combined involvement of these areas. Usually, there is a proliferation of sinusoidal (RE) cells, either as a primary response or one secondary to liver-cell damage.[57] In the case of radiation injury or after administration of such drugs as thorotrast, the sinusoidal cells may be the primary locale of injury. Rarely, sensitizing agents produce an allergic vasculitis which involves the liver. Toxic substances contained in Jamaican

Table 11

SOME DRUGS CAUSING INTRAHEPATIC CHOLESTASIS BY HYPERSENSITIVITY REACTION OR METABOLIC IDIOSYNCRASY

Incidence

> 1 percent

- Chlorpromazine (Thorazine®)
- Mepazine (Pacatal®)
- Prochlorperazine (Compazine®)
- Trifluoperazine (Stelazine®)
- Metahexamide

< 1 percent

- Chlordiazepoxide (Librium®)
- Chlorpropamide (Diabinese®)
- Chlorothiazide (Diuril®)
- Ectylurea (Nostyn®)
- Erythromycin estolate (Ilosone®)
- Methimazole (Tapazole®)
- Promazine hydrochloride (Sparine®)
- Sulfonamides

tea may cause a reaction which primarily affects the hepatic venous system and results in veno-occlusive disease.

Liver-cell damage varies in degree and localization, depending upon the mechanism of the hepatotoxicity and the severity of the reaction. It may be reflected by (1) an alteration in sensitive liver function tests, such as transaminases or BSP, (2) changes in subcellular organelles as observed on the electron microscope, (3) liver-cell necrosis or inflammation noted by light microscopy, and/or (4) clinical evidence of hepatic tenderness and enlargement. The clinical features may be indistinguishable from those described for virus hepatitis (page 61); under these circumstances, the hepatitis may be mild and the cause benign. There may be a fulminant course terminating in acute yellow atrophy, or the process may be long and protracted.

In contrast to patients with liver-cell damage, those with drug-induced intrahepatic cholestasis have laboratory and clinical features characteristic of biliary obstruction. The serum alkaline phosphatase, serum total cholesterol, and BSP may be abnormal prior to development of jaundice. There is evidence of cholestasis, with or without portal inflammation and ductular proliferation, upon light microscopy. Electron microscopy frequently reveals dilatation and atrophy of the microvilli of the bile canaliculi.[67] Lesions of the biliary tract usually subside spontaneously, but the clinical course may be protracted and simulate extrahepatic biliary obstruction and occasionally may lead to all of the manifestations of biliary cirrhosis.[68]

CLINICAL CONSIDERATIONS

A listing of drugs known to have been associated with jaundice may be misleading. The incidence may be extremely low; one antibiotic, for example, has been associated with one case in about every million courses of therapy. Furthermore, the practicing physician must balance the potential risks against the severity of the illness and the likelihood of therapeutic success from the drug in question. In general, however, one would have to consider patients with an allergic background as being especially vulnerable. In addition, drugs with a high incidence of sensitivity reactions should be avoided in patients with preexisting hepatic damage.

Differentiation of drug-induced liver injury from that due to other mechanisms is difficult and may be impossible. Skin tests for sensitivity, unfortunately, are not useful. The presence of coexisting hypersensitivity reactions, such as skin eruptions, angioneurotic edema, or certain hematologic abnormalities, should also arouse suspicion of possible hepatotoxicity.

Besides determining whether liver damage is due to drugs, the physician must also meticulously watch for the development of hepatotoxicity in patients who are receiving drugs. The following approach has been used at the Jersey City Medical Center in patients given a new drug or a drug known to produce toxic or hypersensitivity reactions in the liver:

1. Base-line measurements of liver size and liver function tests are obtained, including transaminases, cephalin flocculation, and plasma removal of BSP. When new drugs are screened, a base-line liver biopsy is obtained, the percentage disappearance rate of BSP is calculated, and thirty and forty-minute levels of the dye are measured. For this purpose, specimens are obtained at five-minute intervals for one hour after injection of 5 mg. of the dye per Kg. of body weight.

2. Studies are repeated at intervals of seven to ten days in the absence of change in liver size, development of hepatic tenderness, or icterus.

3. In the event the patient develops *jaundice*, the drug is discontinued, and studies (previously discussed) are obtained which are necessary to determine the mechanism of hyperbilirubinemia. If intrahepatic cholestasis is present following the use of a drug *not* known to produce this abnormality, the clinician may wish to readminister the drug after hyperbilirubinemia subsides in order to document a cause-and-effect relationship. If cholestasis results from use of an essential therapeutic agent, the clinician may consider readministering the drug in reduced dosage.

4. In cases in which there is a development of *abnormal liver function tests* (*BSP, transaminases, cephalin flocculation*) in the absence of jaundice, the drug is discontinued until the liver function tests return to normal. A drug not known to produce hepatotoxicity may be readministered and the studies repeated. If the drug is known to produce hepatotoxicity regularly, it usually is not readministered.

CONCLUDING REMARKS

This brief review attests to the phenomenal progress made during the past few decades in evaluating the many functions of the liver in health and disease. By using available biochemical, physiologic, morphologic, and radiologic technics, the clinician may now assess the functional status of the hepatic circulatory system, biliary network, reticuloendothelial cells, and liver cells. This approach has permitted the development and objective assessment of preventive and therapeutic measures which should eventually reduce morbidity and mortality of liver disease. Thus, delineation of the role of alcoholism, malnutrition, infective agents, and hepatotoxic drugs in hepatic disease provides a basis for its prevention. More intelligent therapy is possible when these methods are applied to the problems presented by a specific patient.

Current research will further increase our diagnostic ability. Important additional advances should include development of accurate measurements of hepatic blood flow at the bedside, more facile differentiation of intrahepatic and extrahepatic biliary obstruction, development of a practical method for identifying the hepatitis virus, and improvement in current technics for recognizing and delineating factors which interfere with hepatic regeneration. Such additions, hopefully, will lead to the discovery of other effective therapeutic measures and ultimately permit the early recognition, treatment, and cure of hepatic disorders.

APPENDIX

*Tests Generally Available for Diagnostic Study of Patients with Liver Disease**

(Based on current routines at the Jersey City Medical Center†)

Test	*Normal Values*
I. Biochemical studies	
A. Bilirubin	
Direct serum bilirubin	0.1-0.3 mg. per 100 ml.
Total serum bilirubin	0.3-0.5 mg. per 100 ml.
Urine bilirubin	Absent
Urine urobilinogen	Present (1:20)
B. BSP removal	
30-minute ⎫ retention	0-12%
45-minute ⎭	0-5%
Percentage disappearance rate	11-15 mg. per minute
C. Serum alkaline phosphatase	2-5 Bodansky units
D. Total serum cholesterol	180-250 mg. per 100 ml.
Cholesterol esters	60% of total
E. Proteins	
Total serum protein	7.0-7.5 Gm. per 100 ml.
Paper electrophoresis	
Albumin	63-69%
Alpha-1 globulin	3.9-7.3%
Alpha-2 globulin	5.4-8.0%
Beta globulin	6.9-11.8%
Gamma globulin	9.8-20.3%
F. Prothrombin time	Normal
Response of abnormal prothrombin time to vitamin K	Return to normal

*Results of the tests can be properly interpreted only if the clinician is aware of the normal range of values, knows of potential technical errors, and can relate results to clinical features. Normal values should be established for each hospital, and periodic reassessment should be required for accuracy. Serial tests are desirable to provide maximum information.

†These tests are supplemented by hematologic studies when there is an anemia or a hemorrhagic tendency, by metabolic studies for increased hepatic iron, by electrolyte studies when fluid accumulation or renal dysfunction is suspected, and by bacteriologic studies for possible infections.

G. Cephalin flocculation

0-1+

H. Thymol turbidity

0-4 units

  I. Serum enzymes
    Serum glutamic pyruvic transaminase
    Serum glutamic oxalacetic transaminase
    Lactic dehydrogenase

10-40 units
10-40 units
100-350 Berger-Brody units per ml.

  J. Arterial blood ammonia

20-50 μg. per ml.

K. Nucleogenic vitamins
  Serum folic acid
  Serum vitamin B_{12}

6-8 μg. per ml.
200-800 $\mu\mu$g. per ml.

II. Physiologic studies

A. Splenic pulp pressure

8-10 mm. Hg

B. Wedged hepatic vein pressure

6-8 mm. Hg

C. Estimated hepatic blood flow with
  use of indocyanine green

500-800 ml. per sq. M. of body surface per min.

III. Radiologic studies

A. Splenoportogram

Fine vascular pattern extending to surface of liver;
  collaterals not evident

B. Cholecystography and
  cholangiography

Visualization of gall bladder and
  common bile duct without stones

C. Photoscan (I^{131} rose bengal)

Homogeneous density; linear projection in
  midclavicular line—15 $\pm$ 2 cm.

IV. Morphologic studies

A. Light microscopy

Portal and central areas without fibrosis, fat,
  evidence of bile-duct proliferation, bile stasis,
  infiltration, blood stasis, iron, parasites, etc.

B. Electron microscopy

Intact mitochondria, endoplasmic reticula,
  lysosomes, Golgi apparatus, bile canaliculi

C. In-vitro DNA synthesis (tritiated
  thymidine incorporation)

2-3 labeled nuclei per 10,000 liver cells

V. Miscellaneous

A. Esophagoscopy

No evidence of varices

B. Electroencephalography

Normal form, frequency, and amplitude of waves

BIBLIOGRAPHY

1. Libby, W.: The History of Medicine, p. 42. New York: Houghton Mifflin Company, 1922.

2. Long, E. R.: A History of Pathology, p. 176. Baltimore: The Williams & Wilkins Company, 1928.

3. Rappaport, A. M.: Acinar Units and the Pathophysiology of the Liver, in The Liver: Morphology, Biochemistry, Physiology (edited by Ch. Rouiller), Vol. 1, p. 265. New York: Academic Press, Inc., 1963.

4. Naftalis, J., and Leevy, C. M.: Clinical Estimation of Liver Size, Am. J. Digest. Dis., n.s., *8*:236, 1963.

5. Bean, W. B.: The Cutaneous Arterial Spider: A Survey, Medicine, *24*:243, 1945.

6. Groisser, V. W., DiBianco, J., Nissenbaum, G., and Attia, A.: Diagnostic Advances in the Study of Gastrointestinal Bleeding: Experience with a New Device (Diagnostotube) for the Localization of Upper GI Bleeding and the Application of Cinefibergastroscopy in the Study of Bleeding Lesions, paper presented at the First Fall Meeting of the American College of Physicians, Detroit, November 21-23, 1963 (abstr. in Ann. Int. Med., *60*:324 [February], 1964).

7. Davidson, C. S.: Hepatic Coma, in Diseases of the Liver (edited by L. Schiff), p. 234. Philadelphia: J. B. Lippincott Company, 1963.

8. Challenger, F., and Walshe, J. M.: Fœtor Hepaticus, Lancet, *1*:1239, 1955.

9. White, T. J., Leevy, C. M., Brusca, A. M., and Gnassi, A. M.: The Liver in Congestive Heart Failure, Am. Heart J., *49*:250, 1955.

10. Palmerio, C., Zetterstrom, B., Shammash, J., Euchbaum, E., Frank, E., and Fine, J.: Denervation of the Abdominal Viscera for the Treatment of Traumatic Shock, New England J. Med., *269*:709, 1963.

11. Leevy, C. M., Cherrick, G. R., and Davidson, C. S.: Portal Hypertension, New England J. Med., *262*:397, 1960.

12. Bras, G., and McLean, E.: Toxic Factors in Veno-Occlusive Disease, Ann. New York Acad. Sc., *111*:392, 1963.

13. Waldstein, S. S., and Arcilla, R. A.: Measurement of Hepatic Blood Flow by Clearance Methods, Am. J. Digest. Dis., n.s., *3*:137, 1958.

14. Leevy, C. M.: Dye Extraction by the Liver, in Progress in Liver Diseases (edited by H. Popper and F. Schaffner), Vol. 1, p. 174. New York: Grune & Stratton, Inc., 1961.

15. Henning, N., and Demling, L.: Blood Flow in the Liver, in Progress in Liver Diseases (edited by H. Popper and F. Schaffner), Vol. 1, p. 162. New York: Grune & Stratton, Inc., 1961.

16. Bradley, S. E., Ingelfinger, F. J., Bradley, G. P., and Curry, J. J.: The Estimation of Hepatic Blood Flow in Man, J. Clin. Invest., *24*:890, 1945.

17. Combes, B.: Estimation of Hepatic Blood Flow in Man and in Dogs by I^{131}-Labeled Rose Bengal, J. Lab. & Clin. Med., *56*:537, 1960.

18. Cherrick, G. R., Stein, S. W., Leevy, C. M., and Davidson, C. S.: Indocyanine Green: Observations on Its Physical Properties, Plasma Decay, and Hepatic Extraction, J. Clin. Invest., *39*:592, 1960.

19. Hansen, A. T., Tygstrup, N., and Winkler, K.: Determination of the Hepatic Blood Flow by Galactose, Danish M. Bull., *1*:146, 1954.

20. Shaldon, S., Chiandussi, L., Guevara, L., Caesar, J., and Sherlock, S.: The Estimation of Hepatic Blood Flow and Intrahepatic Shunted Blood Flow by Colloidal Heat-Denatured Human Serum Albumin Labeled with I^{131}, J. Clin. Invest., *40*:1346, 1961.

21. Leevy, C. M., Mendenhall, C. L., Lesko, W., and Howard, M. M.: Estimation of Hepatic Blood Flow with Indocyanine Green, J. Clin. Invest., *41*:1169, 1962.

22. Iber, F. L., Kerr, D. N. S., Dölle, W., and Sherlock, S.: Measurement of Blood Flow in the Collateral Vessels of the Portal Vein; Preliminary Results of a New Method, J. Clin. Invest., *39*:1201, 1960.

23. Leevy, C. M., and Gliedman, M. L.: Practical and Research Value of Hepatic-Vein Catheterization, New England J. Med., *258:*696 and 738, 1958.

24. Schlant, R. C., Galambos, J. T., Shuford, W. H., Rawls, W. J., Winter, T. S., and Edwards, F. K.: The Clinical Usefulness of Wedge Hepatic Venography, Am. J. Med., *35:*343, 1963.

25. White, T. J., Wallace, R. B., Gnassi, A. M., Kemp, N. F., Price, H. P., and Leevy, C. M.: Hepatic Abnormalities in Congestive Heart Failure: Needle Biopsy Studies, Circulation, *3:*501, 1951.

26. Palmer, E. D.: Budd-Chiari Syndrome (Occlusion of the Hepatic Veins): Seven Cases, Ann. Int. Med., *41:*261, 1954.

27. Keiding, N. R.: Differentiation into Three Fractions of the Serum Alkaline Phosphatase and the Behavior of the Fractions in Disease of Bone and Liver, Scandinav. J. Clin. & Lab. Invest., *11:*106, 1959.

28. Schaffner, F., Popper, H., and Perez, V.: Changes in Bile Canaliculi Produced by Norethandrolone: Electron Microscopic Study of Human and Rat Liver, J. Lab. & Clin. Med., *56:*623, 1960.

29. Ghadimi, H., and Sass-Kortsak, A.: Evaluation of the Radioactive Rose-Bengal Test for the Differential Diagnosis of Obstructive Jaundice in Infants, New England J. Med., *265:*351, 1961.

30. Bolt, R. J., Dillon, R. S., and Pollard, H. M.: Interference with Bilirubin Excretion by a Gall-Bladder Dye (Bunamiodyl), New England J. Med., *265:*1043, 1961.

31. Wennberg, J. E., Okun, R., Hinman, E. J., Northcutt, R. C., Griep, R. J., and Walker, W. G.: Renal Toxicity of Oral Cholecystographic Media, J.A.M.A., *186:*461, 1963.

32. Schaffner, F., Barka, T., and Popper, H.: Hepatic Mesenchymal Cell Reaction in Liver Disease, Exper. & Molecular Path., *2:*419, 1963.

33. MacDonald, R. A.: Pathogenesis of Nutritional Cirrhosis, Arch. Int. Med., *110:*424, 1962.

34. Benacerraf, B., Biozzi, G., Halpern, B. N., Stiffel, C., and Mouton, D.: Phagocytosis of Heat-Denatured Human Serum Albumin Labelled with ^{131}I and Its Use as a Means of Investigating Liver Blood Flow, Brit. J. Exper. Path., *38:*35, 1957.

35. Iio, M., and Wagner, H. N., Jr.: Studies of the Reticuloendothelial System (RES). I. Measurement of the Phagocytic Capacity of the RES in Man and Dog, J. Clin. Invest., *42:*417, 1963.

36. Salky, N. K., Di Luzio, N. R., P'Pool, D. B., and Sutherland, A. J.: Evaluation of Reticuloendothelial Function in Man, J.A.M.A., *187:*744 (March 7), 1964.

37. Cohen, S., Ohta, G., Singer, E. J., and Popper, H.: Immunocytochemical Study of Gamma Globulin in Liver in Hepatitis and Postnecrotic Cirrhosis, J. Exper. Med., *111:*285, 1960.

38. Leevy, C. M.: In Vitro Studies of Hepatic DNA Synthesis in Percutaneous Liver Biopsy Specimens, J. Lab. & Clin. Med., *61:*761, 1963.

39. Ratnoff, O. D.: Hemostatic Mechanisms in Liver Disease, M. Clin. North America, *47:*721, 1963.

40. Quick, A. J., Stanley-Brown, M., and Bancroft, F. W.: A Study of the Coagulation Defect in Hemophilia and in Jaundice, Am. J. M. Sc., *190:*501, 1935.

41. Hanger, F. M.: The Meaning of Liver Function Tests, Am. J. Med., *16:*565, 1954.

42. Maclagan, N. F., and Bunn, D.: Flocculation Tests with Electrophoretically Separated Serum Proteins, Biochem. J., *41:*580, 1947.

43. Maclagan, N. F.: The Thymol Turbidity Test as an Indicator of Liver Dysfunction, Brit. J. Exper. Path., *25:*234, 1944.

44. Wróblewski, F.: Serum Enzyme Alterations in Diseases of the Liver and Biliary Tract, M. Clin. North America, *44:*699, 1960.

45. Dixon, M., and Webb, E. C.: Enzymes, p. 19. New York: Academic Press, Inc., 1958.

46. Jones, P. N., Mills, E. H., and Capps, R. B.: The Effect of Liver Disease on Serum Vitamin B_{12} Concentrations, J. Lab. & Clin. Med., *49:*910, 1957.

47. Leevy, C. M., Chey, W. Y., Arts, P. A., Mendenhall, C. L., and Howard, M. M.: Protein Tolerance in Liver Disease, Am. J. Clin. Nutrition, *10:*46, 1962.

48. Glomset, J. A.: The Mechanism of the Plasma Cholesterol Esterification Reaction: Plasma Fatty Acid Transferase, Biochim. et biophys. acta, *65:*128, 1962.

49. Schaffner, F., Loebel, A., Weiner, H. A., and Barka, T.: Hepatocellular Cytoplasmic Changes in Acute Alcoholic Hepatitis, J.A.M.A., *183:*343, 1963.

50. Fouts, J. R., and Plaa, G. L.: Hepatic Function and Drug Actions, Biochem. Clin., *3:*123, 1964.

51. Leevy, C. M., and Emmert, J. A.: Problems in the Differential Diagnosis of Jaundice, Rev. Gastroenterology, *20:*422, 1953.

52. Cori, G. T.: Glycogen Structure and Enzyme Deficiencies in Glycogen Storage Disease, Harvey Lectures, Series 48, p. 145, 1952-1953.

53. Isselbacher, K. J., Anderson, E. A., and Kalckar, H. M.: Demonstration of the Specific Enzymatic Defect in Galactosemia, J. Clin. Invest., *35:*714, 1956.

54. Davis, W. D., Jr., and Arrowsmith, W. R.: The Effect of Repeated Phlebotomies in Hemochromatosis: Report of Three Cases, J. Lab. & Clin. Med., *39:*526, 1952.

55. Popper, H., and Schaffner, F.: Fine Structural Changes of the Liver, Ann. Int. Med., *59:*674, 1963.

56. Summerskill, W. H. J., Wolfe, S. J., and Davidson, C. S.: The Metabolism of Ammonia and α-Keto-Acids in Liver Disease and Hepatic Coma, J. Clin. Invest., *36:*361, 1957.

57. Leevy, C. M.: Observations on the Effect of Drug-Induced Injury on Hepatic DNA Synthesis in Experimental Animals and Man, Ann. New York Acad. Sc., *104:*939, 1963.

58. Leevy, C. M., Zinke, M. R., and Chey, W. Y.: Observations on the Distribution of C^{14} Oxytetracycline in Man, Antibiotics Annual, p. 258, 1958-1959.

59. Wheeler, H. O., Meltzer, J. I., and Bradley, S. E.: Biliary Transport and Hepatic Storage of Sulfobromophthalein Sodium in the Unanesthetized Dog, in Normal Man, and in Patients with Hepatic Disease, J. Clin. Invest., *39:*1131, 1960.

60. Peterson, R. E.: Adrenocortical Steroid Metabolism and Adrenal Cortical Function in Liver Disease, J. Clin. Invest., *39:*320, 1960.

61. Osserman, E. F., and Takatsuki, K.: The Plasma Proteins in Liver Disease, M. Clin. North America, *47:*679, 1963.

62. Laidlaw, J., Read, A. E., and Sherlock, S.: Morphine Tolerance in Hepatic Cirrhosis, Gastroenterology, *40:*389, 1961.

63. Leevy, C. M., Tornow, A., Greenberg, P., and Zinke, M.: Observations on the Mode of Action and Clinical Effects of Chlorpropamide in Diabetes Mellitus, Ann. New York Acad. Sc., *74:*725, 1959.

64. Leevy, C. M., George, W., Lesko, W., Deysine, M., Abbott, C. C., and Halligan, E. J.: Observations on Hepatic Oxygen Metabolism in Man, J.A.M.A., *178:*565, 1961.

65. Drill, V. A.: Pharmacology of Hepatotoxic Agents, Ann. New York Acad. Sc., *104:*858, 1963.

66. Zimmerman, H. J.: Clinical and Laboratory Manifestations of Hepatotoxicity, Ann. New York Acad. Sc., *104:*954, 1963.

67. Popper, H., Schaffner, F., Rubin, E., Barka, T., and Paronetto, F.: Mechanisms of Intrahepatic Cholestasis in Drug-Induced Hepatic Injury, Ann. New York Acad. Sc., *104:*988, 1963.

68. Leevy, C. M.: Intrahepatic Cholestasis, Am. J. Surg., *97:*132, 1959.

SUPPLEMENTARY REFERENCES

I. Laboratory Diagnosis of Liver Disease:

Deren, J. J., Williams, L. A., Muench, H., Chalmers, T., and Zamcheck, N.: Comparative Study of Four Methods of Determining Alkaline Phosphatase, New England J. Med., *270*:1277 (June 11), 1964.

Zieve, L., and Hill, E.: An Evaluation of Factors Influencing the Discriminative Effectiveness of a Group of Liver Function Tests. IV. Nature of the Interrelationships among Hepatic Tests in Cirrhosis, Gastroenterology, *28*:914, 1955.

Zieve, L., Hill, E., and Hanson, M.: An Evaluation of Factors Influencing the Discriminative Effectiveness of a Group of Liver Function Tests. VI. Nature of the Interrelationships among Hepatic Tests in Viral Hepatitis, Gastroenterology, *28*:943, 1955.

II. Photoscans in Diagnosis of Liver Disease:

Caroli, J., and Ricordeau, P.: Value of Peritoneoscopy and Peritoneoscopic Photography in Color and of Scintillography in the Diagnosis of Liver Diseases, in Progress in Liver Disease (edited by H. Popper and F. Schaffner), Vol. 1, p. 296. New York: Grune & Stratton, Inc., 1961.

Gollin, F. F., Sims, J. L., and Caméron, J. R.: Liver Scanning and Liver Function Tests, J.A.M.A., *187*:111 (January 11), 1964.

Nagler, W., Bender, M. A., and Blau, M.: Radioisotope Photoscanning of Liver, Gastroenterology, *44*:36, 1963.

Sorensen, L. B.: Radioisotope Scanning in the Diagnosis of Liver Disease, Biochem. Clin., *3*:47, 1964.

Wagner, H. N., Jr., McAfee, J. G., and Mozley, J. M.: Diagnosis of Liver Disease by Radioisotope Scanning, Arch. Int. Med., *107*:324, 1961.

III. Physiology of the Hepatic Circulation:

Bradley, S. E.: The Circulation and the Liver, Gastroenterology, *44*:403, 1963.

Brauer, R. W.: Liver Circulation and Function, Physiol. Rev., *43*:115, 1963.

Cocco, T. B., Judy, K. H., and Leevy, C. M.: Observations on Intrahepatic Vascular Regulation in Portal Hypertension, Ann. Surg., *158*:109, 1963.

Leevy, C. M., tenHove, W., and Howard, M.: Mesenchymal-Cell Proliferation in Liver Disease of the Alcoholic, J.A.M.A., *187*:598 (February 22), 1964.

Schaffner, F., and Popper, H.: Capillarization of Hepatic Sinusoids in Man, Gastroenterology, *44*:239, 1963.

IV. Splenoportography:

DeWeese, M. S., Figley, M. M., Fry, W. J., Rapp, R., and Smith, H. L.: Clinical Appraisal of Percutaneous Splenoportography, A.M.A. Arch. Surg., *75*:423, 1957.

Panke, W. F., Bradley, E. G., Moreno, A. H., Ruzicka, F. F., Jr., and Rousselot, L. M.: Technique, Hazards and Usefulness of Percutaneous Splenic Portography, J.A.M.A., *169*:1032, 1959.

Turner, M. D., Sherlock, S., and Steiner, R. E.: Splenic Venography and Intrasplenic Pressure Measurement in the Clinical Investigation of the Portal Venous System, Am. J. Med., *23*:846, 1957.

V. Bilirubin Metabolism and Jaundice:

Arias, I. M.: Chronic Unconjugated Hyperbilirubinemia without Overt Signs of Hemolysis in Adolescents and Adults, J. Clin. Invest., *41*:2233, 1962.

Billing, B. H., and Lathe, G. H.: Bilirubin Metabolism in Jaundice, Am. J. Med., *24*:111, 1958.

Klatskin, G.: Bile Pigment Metabolism, Ann. Rev. Med., *12:*211, 1961.

Lester, R., and Schmid, R.: Bilirubin Metabolism, New England J. Med., *270:*779 (April 9), 1964.

Sass-Kortsak, A., Macdougall, L. G., Ghadimi, H., and Cherniak, M. M.: Differential Diagnosis of Regurgitation Jaundice in Early Infancy, Ann. New York Acad. Sc., *111:*422, 1963.

Sherlock, S.: Jaundice, Brit. M. J., *1:*1359, 1962.

Watson, C. J.: The Importance of the Fractional Serum Bilirubin Determination in Clinical Medicine, Ann. Int. Med., *45:*351, 1956.

VI. Dye Extraction by Liver:

Brent, R. L., and Geppert, L. J.: The Use of Radioactive Rose Bengal in the Evaluation of Infantile Jaundice, A.M.A. J. Dis. Child., *98:*720, 1959.

Englert, E., Jr., Burrows, B. A., and Ingelfinger, F. J.: Differential Analysis of the Stages of Hepatic Excretory Function with Gamma Emitting Isotopes, J. Lab. & Clin. Med., *56:*181, 1960.

Fauvert, R. E., Weber, J., and Benhamou, J.: Bromsulphalein Fractional Clearance, Biochem. Clin., *3:*39, 1964.

Leevy, C. M., Bender, J., Silverberg, M., and Naylor, J.: Physiology of Dye Extraction by the Liver: Comparative Studies of Sulfobromophthalein and Indocyanine Green, Ann. New York Acad. Sc., *111:*161, 1963.

Mendenhall, C. L., and Leevy, C. M.: False-Negative Bromsulfalein Tests, New England J. Med., *264:*431, 1961.

VII. Cholecystography and Cholangiography:

Cuniff, C. L., Dolan, M. A., and Leevy, C. M.: Cholecystography in Portal Cirrhosis without Jaundice, Gastroenterology, *25:*557, 1953.

Kantor, H. G., Evans, J. A., and Glenn, F.: Cholangiography: A Critical Analysis, A.M.A. Arch. Surg., *70:*237, 1955.

Kaplan, A. A., Traitz, J. J., Mitchel, S. D., and Block, A. L.: Percutaneous Transhepatic Cholangiography, Ann. Int. Med., *54:*856, 1961.

Santos, M., Figueroa, L., and López, O.: Percutaneous Transhepatic Cholangiography in the Diagnosis of Posthepatic Jaundice, Surgery, *48:*295, 1960.

VIII. Coagulation Disturbances in Liver Disease:

Finkbiner, R. B., McGovern, J. J., Goldstein, R., and Bunker, J. P.: Coagulation Defects in Liver Disease and Response to Transfusion during Surgery, Am. J. Med., *26:*199, 1959.

Mindrum, G., and Glueck, H. I.: Plasma Prothrombin in Liver Disease: Its Clinical and Prognostic Significance, Ann. Int. Med., *50:*1370, 1959.

Rapaport, S. I., Ames, S. B., Mikkelsen, S., and Goodman, J. R.: Plasma Clotting Factors in Chronic Hepatocellular Disease, New England J. Med., *263:*278, 1960.

IX. Serum Enzyme Changes in Liver Disease:

Gutman, A. B.: Serum Alkaline Phosphatase Activity in Diseases of the Skeletal and Hepatobiliary Systems: A Consideration of the Current Status, Am. J. Med., *27:*875, 1959.

Hill, B. R.: Further Studies of the Fractionation of Lactic Dehydrogenase of Blood, Ann. New York Acad. Sc., *75:*304, 1958.

Iber, F. L., Greene, R., and Harvey, A. M.: Serum Alkaline Phosphatase in Infiltrative Diseases of the Liver, Biochem. Clin., *3:*177, 1964.

Pineda, E. P., Goldbarg, J. A., Banks, B. M., and Rutenburg, A. M.: Serum Leucine Aminopeptidase in Pancreatic and Hepatobiliary Diseases, Gastroenterology, *38:*698, 1960.

X. Blood Ammonia and Hepatic Encephalopathy:

Butt, H. R., and Summerskill, W. H. J.: Hepatic Coma, in Progress in Liver Disease (edited by H. Popper and F. Schaffner), Vol. 1, p. 109. New York: Grune & Stratton, Inc., 1961.

Chalmers, T. C.: Pathogenesis and Treatment of Hepatic Failure, New England J. Med., *263*:23, 1960.

Conn, H. O.: Ammonia Tolerance in Liver Disease, J. Lab. & Clin. Med., *55*:855, 1960.

Gabuzda, G. J., Phillips, G. B., and Davidson, C. S.: Reversible Toxic Manifestations in Patients with Cirrhosis of the Liver Given Cation-Exchange Resins, New England J. Med., *246*:124, 1952.

Sherlock, S.: Pathogenesis and Management of Hepatic Coma, Am. J. Med., *24*:805, 1958.

XI. Portal Hypertension and Bleeding Varices:

Child, C. G., III, and Turcotte, J. G.: Surgery and Portal Hypertension, in The Liver and Portal Hypertension (edited by C. G. Child III), p. 1. Philadelphia: W. B. Saunders Company, 1964.

Leevy, C. M.: Portal Hypertension and Bleeding, in Modern Treatment (edited by R. B. Capps), Vol. 1, p. 462. New York: Paul B. Hoeber, Inc., 1964.

Reynolds, T. B., Balfour, D. C., Jr., Levinson, D. C., Mikkelsen, W. P., and Pattison, A. C.: Comparison of Wedged Hepatic Vein Pressure with Portal Vein Pressure in Human Subjects with Cirrhosis, J. Clin. Invest., *34*:213, 1955.

Taylor, W. J., and Myers, J. D.: Occlusive Hepatic Venous Catheterization in the Study of the Normal Liver, Cirrhosis of the Liver and Noncirrhotic Portal Hypertension, Circulation, *13*:368, 1956.

XII. Fluid and Electrolyte Disturbances and Ascites:

Baldus, W. P., Feichter, R. N., Summerskill, W. H. J., Hunt, J. C., and Wakim, K. G.: The Kidney in Cirrhosis. II. Disorders of Renal Function, Ann. Int. Med., *60*:366 (March), 1964.

Hanger, F. M. (Moderator): Pathogenesis and Management of Ascites, transcription of a panel meeting, Bull. New York Acad. Med., *39*:238, 1963.

Howard, M. M., and Leevy, C. M.: Management of Ascites, Arch. Int. Med., *112*:702, 1963.

Papper, S.: Role of the Kidney in Laennec's Cirrhosis of the Liver, Medicine, *37*:299, 1958.

XIII. Clinicopathologic Correlations:

Baggenstoss, A. H.: Postnecrotic Cirrhosis: Morphology, Etiology and Pathogenesis, in Progress in Liver Disease (edited by H. Popper and F. Schaffner), Vol. 1, p. 14. New York: Grune & Stratton, Inc., 1961.

Gall, E. A.: Posthepatitic, Postnecrotic, and Nutritional Cirrhosis: A Pathologic Analysis, Am. J. Path., *36*:241, 1960.

Landing, B. H.: Lesions of the Liver in Hereditary Metabolic Diseases, Ann. New York Acad. Sc., *111*:399, 1963.

Leevy, C. M.: Fatty Liver: A Study of 270 Patients with Biopsy Proven Fatty Liver and a Review of the Literature, Medicine, *41*:249, 1962.

Leevy, C. M.: Hepatic DNA Synthesis and Regeneration, Biochem. Clin., *3*:109, 1964.

Leevy, C. M., Gellene, R., and Ning, M.: Primary Liver Cancer in Cirrhosis of the Alcoholic, Ann. New York Acad. Sc., *114*:1026 (April 2), 1964.

Novikoff, A. B., and Essner, E.: The Liver Cell: Some New Approaches to Its Study, Am. J. Med., *29*:102, 1960.

Popper, H., Rubin, E., Krus, S., and Schaffner, F.: Postnecrotic Cirrhosis in Alcoholics, Gastroenterology, *39:*669, 1960.

Rouiller, Ch., and Jézéquel, A.-M.: Electron Microscopy of the Liver, in The Liver (edited by Ch. Rouiller), Vol. 1, p. 195. New York: Academic Press, Inc., 1963.

Rubin, E., Schaffner, F., and Popper, H.: Localization of the Basic Injury in Primary Biliary Cirrhosis, J.A.M.A., *183:*331, 1963.

Smetana, H. F.: The Histopathology of Drug-Induced Liver Disease, Ann. New York Acad. Sc., *104:*821, 1963.

XIV. Biochemical Analyses of Liver Tissue in Hepatic Disease:

Baker, H., Frank, O., Ziffer, H., Goldfarb, S., Leevy, C. M., and Sobotka, H.: Effect of Hepatic Disease on Liver B-Complex Vitamin Titers, Am. J. Clin. Nutrition, *14:*1 (January), 1964.

de Duve, C., and Berthet, J.: The Use of Differential Centrifugation in the Study of Tissue Enzymes, Internat. Rev. Cytol., *3:*225, 1954.

Henley, K. S., Wiggins, H. S., Pollard, H. M., and Dullaert, E.: The Transaminase Content of Parenchymatous Liver Cells, Gastroenterology, *36:*1, 1959.

Moulé, Y., and Chauveau, J.: The Cell Components of the Liver, in The Liver (edited by Ch. Rouiller), Vol. 1, p. 379. New York: Academic Press, Inc., 1963.

Pagliaro, L., Notarbartolo, A., Mannino, V., and Migneco, G.: Reduced Ability of Mitochondria Isolated from Liver Tissue of Patients with Cirrhosis to Synthesize ATP, J. Lab. & Clin. Med., *62:*184, 1963.

XV. Drug-Induced Liver Injury:

Drill, V. A.: Symposium on Toxic Hepatic Injury, Gastroenterology, *38:*786, 1960.

Kalow, W.: Genetic Differences in Drug Metabolism, Ann. New York Acad. Sc., *104:*894, 1963.

Klatskin, G.: Toxic Hepatitis, in Diseases of the Liver (edited by L. Schiff), p. 328. Philadelphia: J. B. Lippincott Company, 1963.

Ticktin, H. E., and Robinson, M. M.: Effects of Some Antimicrobial Agents on the Liver, Ann. New York Acad. Sc., *104:*1080, 1963.

INDEX

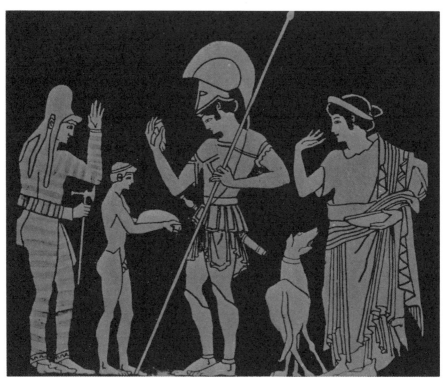

Adrastus leaving for the Theban war consults the liver of a victim
(from a Greek vase painting).